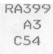

Clinical
Pract
Guidelines

Directions for a New Program

Committee to Advise the Public Health Service
on Clinical Practice Guidelines

Institute of Medicine

Marilyn J. Field and Kathleen N. Lohr, editors

NATIONAL ACADEMY PRESS
Washington, D.C. 1990

ject of this report was approved by the Governing ncil, whose members are drawn from the councils of ences, the National Academy of Engineering, and the Institute The members of the committee responsible for the report were chosen for their special competencies and with regard for appropriate balance.

This report has been reviewed by a group other than the authors according to procedures approved by a Report Review Committee consisting of members of the National Academy of Sciences, the National Academy of Engineering, and the Institute of Medicine.

The Institute of Medicine was chartered in 1970 by the National Academy of Sciences to enlist distinguished members of the appropriate professions in the examination of policy matters pertaining to the health of the public. In this, the Institute acts under both the Academy's 1863 congressional charter responsibility to be an adviser to the federal government and its own initiative in identifying issues of medical care, research, and education.

This project was supported by the Department of Health and Human Services, Contract No. 282-90-0018. The views presented are those of the Institute of Medicine Committee to Advise the Public Health Service on Clinical Practice Guidelines and are not necessarily those of the funding organization. The Andrew W. Mellon Foundation contribution to independent Institute of Medicine funds was also used to support the project.

Library of Congress Catalog Card Number 90-062881
International Standard Book Number 0-309-04346-8
Publication IOM-90-08

Additional copies of this report are available from:

National Academy Press
2101 Constitution Avenue, N.W.
Washington, DC 20418

First Printing, September 1990
Second Printing, November 1991
Third Printing, October 1992
Fourth Printing, February 1993

S-229

Printed in the United States of America

WILLIAM B. STASON, Director, Northeast Health Services, Research & Development Field Program, Veterans Administration Medical Center, West Roxbury, Massachusetts

MICHAEL A. STOCKER, Executive Vice President, U.S. Healthcare, Paramus, New Jersey

JAMES J. STRAIN, Professor and Director, Division of Behavioral Medicine and Consultation Psychiatry, Mt. Sinai School of Medicine, New York, New York

LINDA JOHNSON WHITE, Director, Department of Scientific Policy, American College of Physicians, Philadelphia, Pennsylvania

CONSTANCE M. WINSLOW, Medical Director, Research and Program Development, AEtna Life and Casualty, Hartford, Connecticut

STUDY STAFF

KARL D. YORDY, Director, Division of Health Care Services
MARILYN J. FIELD, Study Co-Director
KATHLEEN N. LOHR, Study Co-Director
MOLLA S. DONALDSON, Senior Staff Officer
THELMA COX, Project Secretary
DONALD TILLER, Administrative Assistant

Acknowledgments

This project was shaped by the work of two earlier Institute of Medicine committees: the Committee on Utilization Management by Third Parties and the Committee to Design a Strategy for Quality Review and Assurance in Medicare. The report of the first committee was issued in October 1989 and the report of the second, in March 1990. Some of the substantive groundwork for this report was laid by an expert panel convened for the quality assurance project to consider desirable characteristics of quality of care indicators. That panel consisted of William A. Causey, Arthur J. Donovan, Leonard S. Dreifus, David M. Eddy, Lesley Fishelman, Sheldon Greenfield, Robert J. Marder, Jane L. Neumann, Bruce Perry, and Ralph Schaffarzick.

Both the utilization management and quality assurance committees made recommendations for further work on the development and use of clinical practice guidelines that led to a project planning meeting in November 1989. The meeting was chaired by Jerome H. Grossman, and the participants were Peter Bouxsein, J. Jarrett Clinton, Arthur J. Donovan, David M. Eddy, Sheldon Greenfield, Clark C. Havighurst, Neil Hollander, Carmault B. Jackson, Jr., John T. Kelly, Marie Michnich, Joel E. Miller, William H. Moncreif, Jr., Charles E. Phelps, William L. Roper, Ralph Schaffarzick, Richard S. Sharpe, Linda Johnson White, and Sally Hart Wilson.

As background for the planning meeting and the study committee, Anne-Marie Audet and Sheldon Greenfield of the Institute for the Advancement of Health and Medical Care of the New England Medical

Center, Inc., conducted a focused survey of prototypical initiatives on clinical practice guidelines. Marilyn Field, study co-director, prepared a background case study of mammography screening guidelines. Dr. Greenfield also made a presentation to the study committee as did Mark R. Chassin of Value Health Sciences. IOM Scholar-in-Residence Patrick Mattingly and Robert Wood Johnson Fellow Philip Goodman provided useful suggestions and information. Stephen King, director of the Forum for Quality and Effectiveness in Health Care, Agency for Health Care Policy and Research, was always helpful in providing necessary information on the agency. In addition, he briefed the study committee at its February and April meetings.

From January through March 1990, Don Tiller kept the study operational by overseeing the work of a series of temporary secretaries until Suzanna Gilbert began work in April. Marilyn Field and Kathleen Lohr had primary responsibility for writing the report with assistance from Molla Donaldson, who also prepared two sets of examples of practice guidelines for the committee's examination. Leah Mazade copyedited the report. The editors also acknowledge the constructive comments of those who reviewed the report under National Research Council procedures.

Contents

Summary

In November 1989, Congress amended the Public Health Service Act to create the Agency for Health Care Policy and Research (AHCPR). Under the terms of Public Law 101-239, this agency has broad responsibilities for supporting research, data development, and other activities that will "enhance the quality, appropriateness, and effectiveness of health care services. . . ." The needs and priorities of the Medicare program are an important but not exclusive focus of the agency.

Many of AHCPR's responsibilities formerly belonged to the National Center for Health Services Research, which the agency replaced, but the emphasis on outcomes and effectiveness research is now considerably stronger. Other functions of the agency are new, in particular those involving a joint public-private enterprise to develop, disseminate, and evaluate practice guidelines under the sponsorship of the agency's Forum for Quality and Effectiveness in Health Care.

Shortly after its creation, AHCPR requested advice from the Institute of Medicine (IOM) on how it might approach these new responsibilities for practice guidelines. The IOM agreed to appoint a study committee that would work quickly to provide technical assistance and advice on definition of terms, specification of key attributes of good guidelines, and certain aspects of planning for implementation and evaluation. This report largely confines itself to these fairly specific and limited tasks. It is not a how-to-do-it manual, a methodology text, a priority-setting exercise, or a primer on guidelines for those seeking an introduction to the subject. The report does, however, aim to encourage more standardization and consistency in

1

guidelines development, whether such development is supported directly by the Forum or is undertaken independently by medical societies and other organizations.

The committee believes that the AHCPR initiative, taken as a whole, has real potential to advance the state of the art for practice guidelines, strengthen the knowledge base for health care practice, and, hence, improve the appropriateness and effectiveness of health care. One objective of this report is to encourage realistic expectations about this potential by building a broader understanding of the difficult but important steps needed to move toward the goals for practice guidelines stated in P.L. 101-239, or, as it is also called, the Omnibus Budget Reconciliation Act of 1989 (OBRA 89).

CONTEXT

The committee began its work with an understanding that the legislation establishing AHCPR is one consequence of accumulated public and private frustrations about the perceived health and economic consequences of inappropriate medical care. These frustrations and perceptions stem from many sources including ceaselessly escalating health care costs, wide variations in medical practice patterns, evidence that some health services are of little or no value, and claims that various kinds of financial, educational, and organizational incentives can reduce inappropriate utilization.

The combination of high expenditures and doubts about the value of that spending explains policymakers' interest in improving the scope and application of knowledge about what works and what does not work in medical care—and at what price. AHCPR is supporting an extensive agenda of outcomes and effectiveness research. In fact, the major part of the agency's work involves expanding the scope of knowledge rather than applying it. Of AHCPR's appropriation of nearly $100 million for fiscal year 1990, it planned to obligate around $2 million for the Forum's work on practice guidelines, compared with more than $30 million for outcomes research. Still, the agency's responsibilities for practice guidelines reflect congressional recognition of the practical need for ways to translate knowledge into patient and practitioner decisions that improve the value the nation receives for its health care spending.

More generally, the creation of a practice guidelines function within AHCPR can be seen as part of a significant cultural shift, a move away from unexamined reliance on professional judgment toward more structured support and accountability for such judgment. Reflecting the first element of this shift, guidelines are intended to assist practitioners and patients in making health care decisions; reflecting the second aspect, they are to serve as a foundation for instruments to evaluate practitioner and health system performance.

OVERVIEW OF PRACTICE GUIDELINES INITIATIVES

Public and private activities related to practice guidelines can be conceptualized, ideally, as having three basic stages: development, intervention, and evaluation. The second and third stages should—again ideally—involve feedback loops to the first stage to prompt the revision of guidelines when omissions, technical obsolescence, or other problems with a set of guidelines are identified. Guidelines are thus dynamic, not static. They reflect the interplay of scientific and technological progress, real-world organizational pressures, and changes in social values. To date, most government and other initiatives emphasize the first of the three stages, the development of guidelines.

PUBLIC INITIATIVES

Under OBRA 89, Congress created within AHCPR the Office of the Forum for Quality and Effectiveness in Health Care. The Forum must "arrange for" the development and periodic review and updating of

(1) clinically relevant guidelines that may be used by physicians, educators, and health care practitioners to assist in determining how diseases, disorders, and other health conditions can most effectively and appropriately be prevented, diagnosed, treated, and managed clinically; and
(2) standards of quality, performance measures, and medical review criteria through which health care providers and other appropriate entities may assess or review the provision of health care and assure the quality of such care.

The phrase "arrange for" is one key indicator of the extent to which the drafters of OBRA 89 sought to create a public-private enterprise with respect to guidelines development. Their vision was that the Forum would itself develop no guidelines; guidelines were not to be federal creations.

By January 1, 1991, the Forum must arrange for the development of an initial set of guidelines, standards, performance measures, and review criteria for at least three clinical treatments or conditions. The agency is also responsible for updating the guidelines developed under its auspices. Other key provisions of the legislation include the following.

- The Forum can contract with public and nonprofit private organizations to develop and update guidelines, or it can convene expert panels to either develop guidelines or review guidelines developed by contractors.
- The director of the Forum must establish the standards for methods and procedures to be followed by the contractors and expert panels. The guidelines can be pilot-tested.

- Guidelines developed by private organizations independently of the agency program may be adopted by contractors or expert panels if they meet the requirements established by the legislation.
- The director of the Forum is to promote dissemination of guidelines through organizations representing health care providers, health care consumers, peer review organizations, accrediting bodies, and other appropriate entities. In addition, the guidelines must be presented in formats appropriate for use by practitioners, medical educators, and medical care reviewers.
- The Secretary of the Department of Health and Human Services (DHHS) "shall provide for the use of the [initial sets of] guidelines . . . to improve the quality, effectiveness, and appropriateness of care" provided under the Medicare program. Presumably, providing for the use of the guidelines will require that the Health Care Financing Administration (HCFA) and its contracting fiscal intermediaries, carriers, and peer review organizations take steps to incorporate review criteria and other evaluation instruments into their programs for reviewing care provided to Medicare beneficiaries.
- The director of the Forum is to conduct and support evaluations of the impact of guidelines on clinical practice. More specifically, for the guidelines developed by January 1, 1991, the Secretary of DHHS must determine the impact of the initial sets of guidelines on the cost, quality, appropriateness, and effectiveness of medical care provided under the Medicare program and report the results to Congress by January 1, 1993.
- With respect to the research agenda of AHCPR, the director of the Forum is to recommend research projects related to the outcomes of health care, the processes for developing guidelines, and the use of guidelines.

In general, when it examines clinical conditions as potential subjects for guidelines, the agency is instructed to consider how guidelines, standards, performance measures, and review criteria can be expected to (1) improve health for a significant number of individuals, (2) reduce clinically significant variations in services and procedures provided by physicians, and (3) reduce clinically significant variations in the outcomes of health care. Moreover, the administrator of the agency is to consult with the Health Care Financing Administration and ensure that the needs and priorities of the Medicare program are appropriately reflected in the development of guidelines. For the initial three sets of guidelines, the legislation provides more specific selection priorities related to expenditures and services for Medicare beneficiaries.

In addition to the new agency, other agencies of the federal government have related responsibilities. These agencies include the National Institutes of Health (NIH), the U.S. Preventive Services Task Force, and the Health Care Financing Administration and its contracting carriers, fiscal intermediaries, and peer review organizations.

PRIVATE INITIATIVES

Guidelines for clinical practice, broadly defined, are not new. The processes of organized clinical education require various sorts of guidelines, as do the processes of professional licensure, board certification, quality assurance, utilization review, and other aspects of health services administration. However, the interest of the medical community and others in practice guidelines has grown exponentially in recent years. Moreover, there is greater emphasis today on formal procedures and methods for arriving at a widely scrutinized and endorsed consensus.

Among the medical groups involved for some years with the development of guidelines are the American Academy of Family Physicians, the American College of Cardiology, the American College of Physicians, and the American Society of Anesthesiologists. In the research community, the RAND Corporation has pioneered the development of important tools and strategies. Newer initiatives are being undertaken or planned by the American Board of Medical Specialties, the American Medical Association, the Council of Medical Specialty Societies, many individual specialty societies, and the academic medical and health services research community.

Insurers, health maintenance organizations (HMOs), utilization management firms, and similar organizations have not ignored the potential of practice guidelines to serve as a basis for refusing payment for inappropriate care. For example, several years ago, the Blue Cross and Blue Shield Association began its Medical Necessity Project, which worked with researchers and some medical organizations to identify obsolete procedures and set guidelines for the appropriate use of many diagnostic and treatment services. The Health Insurance Association of America recently established a similar function, and the Group Health Association of America has been sponsoring programs on guidelines development. Individual members of each of these associations are involved in additional efforts to develop or adapt guidelines to meet the needs of their different health plans. The activities of dozens of firms supplying utilization management services to health plan sponsors have drawn attention to the quality, scope, and accessibility of the criteria they use to review care on a prospective or concurrent basis.

The guidelines development efforts of private organizations are thus proceeding on many fronts. Some coordinating strategies are emerging, but important problems remain—unexplained conflicts among guidelines, neglected topics, lack of follow-up, and incomplete public disclosure of the evidence, participants, and methods used to develop sets of guidelines. No independent entity exists to certify that guidelines are sound in method and content, and no "national bureau of standards" is available to set standards for methods of guidelines development or their content. The legislation creating AHCPR is one response to some of these problems.

INSTITUTE OF MEDICINE COMMITTEE AND PROJECT

The major immediate goal of this project was to help the Forum prepare to work with contractors or expert panels to meet its January 1991 deadline for developing at least three sets of guidelines. This assistance is also meant to help the Forum assess the soundness of the products (the guidelines) emerging from these contractors or panels. A second IOM project, described at the end of this summary, will develop a practical evaluation instrument for this purpose.

To conduct the study requested by AHCPR, the IOM appointed a committee of experts in January 1990 that met in February and again in April. The committee included practicing physicians, individuals experienced in the development of guidelines, current and potential users of guidelines, and representatives of relevant other disciplines such as nursing, law, and economics. Staff from the Forum attended both committee meetings and received copies of all draft and background materials prepared for the committee.

FINDINGS AND CONCLUSIONS

STATE OF THE ART

The committee arrived at several general observations about the state of the art of practice guidelines development. Most generally, the process of systematic development, implementation, and evaluation of practice guidelines based on rigorous clinical research and soundly generated professional consensus, although progressing, has deficiencies in method, scope, and substance. Conflicts in terminology and technique characterize the field; they are notable for the confusion they create and for what they reflect about differences in values, experiences, and interests among different parties. Public and private development activities are multiplying, but the means for coordinating these efforts to resolve inconsistencies, fill in gaps, track applications and results, and assess the soundness of particular guidelines are limited. Disproportionately more attention is paid to developing guidelines than to implementing or evaluating them. Moreover, efforts to develop guidelines are necessarily constrained by inadequacies in the quality and quantity of scientific evidence on the effectiveness of many services.

AHCPR AND THE FORUM

As a consequence of the above factors, AHCPR and the Forum have, at present, a somewhat restricted foundation for their work. In addition, at least three other variables must be taken into account in estimating what the agency is likely to be able to accomplish early in its guidelines effort. First, although OBRA 89 addresses some concerns about guidelines development, implementation, and evaluation, it appropriately does not describe a precise course of action. The agency will need time to devise and revise practical and defensible approaches to guidelines development.

Second, given that both the function and the organizational units (particularly the Forum) are new to the Department of Health and Human Services, the legislative timetables for guidelines development and, particularly, evaluation are unrealistically short. Moreover, the Forum has few staff to support the new functions, a deficit that is not likely to change in the near term. In the immediate future, these constraints and complications are facts of life; the agency is acting to meet its deadlines in as timely and meaningful a way as possible. Over the longer run, however, the committee hopes that experience with the practicalities of guidelines development will lead Congress and the agency to moderate the development and evaluation timetables or to expand the resources devoted to the tasks, or both.

Third, within the government, meeting the challenge of developing good practice guidelines cannot be solely the responsibility of the Forum. For instance, AHCPR's Medical Treatment Effectiveness Program (MEDTEP) will generate information of immediate importance for practice guidelines. Lacunae in data identified during the guidelines development process should highlight areas that AHCPR can target for research funding. Outside AHCPR, the work of other agencies in the Public Health Service (PHS), most notably NIH's randomized controlled trials, will be essential to the long-term utility of guidelines, especially insofar as those trials include broad measures of outcomes important to patients. Outside the PHS, the agency needs to maintain close links with the Health Care Financing Administration, in part because of provisions of OBRA 89 but more importantly because HCFA's data on the Medicare population (and, to a lesser extent, on the Medicaid population) should be valuable for developing, implementing, and evaluating guidelines.

ROLES OF PUBLIC AND PRIVATE SECTORS

Despite the focus of this study on advice to a federal agency, the committee believes that the government's role in arranging for the development of practice guidelines may in the end be fairly modest. Indeed, the contemporaneous efforts of many different organizations in the private sector may significantly outpace what this one agency can do. The predominance of the private sector should be even greater for guidelines implementation, where most initiative must rest with private organizations and individuals. Even when the government plays the principal role in funding and disseminating guidelines on certain topics or clinical conditions, these guidelines will be tailored or adjusted by providers, health plans, and others to reflect different patient populations, delivery settings, practitioner skills and attitudes, levels of resources, perceptions of risk, and other factors. The committee expects that the processes of guidelines development, implementation, and evaluation will always need to be pursued by both the public and private sectors.

RECOMMENDATIONS: DEFINITIONS

If the Forum is to proceed confidently with its mission, it needs clear and broadly acceptable definitions of four key terms used in OBRA 89: (1) practice guidelines, (2) medical review criteria, (3) standards of quality, and (4) performance measures. Neither the final legislation nor preceding House or Senate bills offered definitions of these particular terms, and the literature on practice guidelines and related topics is characterized by significant diversity in common and professional usage.

This report aims to provide definitions that are—insofar as possible— parsimonious, clear, not tautological, consistent with customary professional and legislative usage, and socially and practically acceptable to important interests. The committee recommends that the agency work with the following definitions.

PRACTICE GUIDELINES are systematically developed statements to assist practitioner and patient decisions about appropriate health care for specific clinical circumstances.

MEDICAL REVIEW CRITERIA are systematically developed statements that can be used to assess the appropriateness of specific health care decisions, services, and outcomes.

STANDARDS OF QUALITY are authoritative statements of (1) minimum levels of acceptable performance or results, (2) excellent levels of performance or results, *or* (3) the range of acceptable performance or results.

PERFORMANCE MEASURES (Provisional) are methods or instruments to estimate or monitor the extent to which the actions of a health care practitioner or provider conform to practice guidelines, medical review criteria, or standards of quality.

The committee recognizes that the definitions will not resolve all arguments over what these and related terms mean, but it does believe that these four statements will bring a degree of badly needed clarity and uniformity to the field. Moreover, these definitions can be used by the Forum and, indeed, have already been incorporated into its work.

One underlying premise highlighted by these definitions is that these four terms are not synonymous. Assisting physicians, nurses, other practitioners, and patients in making decisions (through practice guidelines) is not the same as evaluating practice (using medical review criteria, standards of quality, and performance measures). Therefore, although the definitions may evolve, it is important to underscore that the phrases and concepts are not equivalent and should not be used interchangeably. For various practical or technical reasons, some elements of a set of guidelines may have no corresponding review criteria or other evaluation tools.

Not part of the committee's definition of practice guidelines, but central to its view of the field, is the precept that every set of guidelines should be accompanied by a statement of the strength of the scientific evidence and the expert judgment behind them and by projections of the relevant health and cost outcomes. The committee has not tried to distinguish types or levels of practice guidelines (for example, Levels 1 or 2), although this type of discrimination may be useful.

RECOMMENDATIONS: ATTRIBUTES OF GOOD GUIDELINES

Developing practice guidelines is a challenging task that requires diverse skills ranging from analysis of scientific evidence to management of group decisionmaking to presentation of complex information in understandable forms. To arrange for the development of guidelines by expert panels and contractors, the Forum must be able to state its expectations for the process and then assess the soundness of the resulting products. (OBRA 89 calls this establishing "standards and criteria" for the process. To avoid confusion, this report substitutes the term *attributes* for the statutory language. As described at the end of this summary, the IOM is preparing in provisional form a practical assessment instrument for the agency.)

This report distinguishes between the priorities for selecting particular targets for guidelines and the desirable attributes of guidelines. Priority setting is a crucial but separate task for which OBRA 89 provides guidance.

Drawing on its members' experience and expertise and the work of past IOM committees and other relevant organizations, the committee recommends that the agency use the following eight attributes, properties, or characteristics to instruct expert panels or contractors and to assess their products. The attributes focus on practice guidelines and not on medical review criteria and other tools for evaluating practice. The committee expects this set of attributes to be tested, reassessed, and, if necessary, revised.

VALIDITY: Practice guidelines are valid if, when followed, they lead to the health and cost outcomes projected for them, other things being equal. A prospective assessment of validity will consider the projected health outcomes and costs of alternative courses of action, the relationship between the evidence and recommendations, the substance and quality of the scientific and clinical evidence cited, and the means used to evaluate the evidence.

RELIABILITY/REPRODUCIBILITY: Practice guidelines are reliable and reproducible (1) if—given the same evidence and methods for guidelines development—another set of experts would produce essentially the same statements and (2) if—given the same circumstances—the guidelines are interpreted and applied consistently by practitioners or other appropriate parties. A prospective assessment of reliability may consider the results of independent external reviews and pretests of the guidelines.

CLINICAL APPLICABILITY: Practice guidelines should be as inclusive of appropriately defined patient populations as scientific and clinical evidence and expert judgment permit, and they should explicitly state the populations to which statements apply.

CLINICAL FLEXIBILITY: Practice guidelines should identify the specifically known or generally expected exceptions to their recommendations.

CLARITY: Practice guidelines should use unambiguous language, define terms precisely, and use logical, easy-to-follow modes of presentation.

MULTIDISCIPLINARY PROCESS: Practice guidelines should be developed by a process that includes participation by representatives of key affected groups. Participation may include serving on panels that develop guidelines, providing evidence and viewpoints to the panels, and reviewing draft guidelines.

SCHEDULED REVIEW: Practice guidelines should include statements about when they should be reviewed to determine whether revisions are warranted, given new clinical evidence or changing professional consensus.

DOCUMENTATION: The procedures followed in developing guidelines, the participants involved, the evidence used, the assumptions and rationales accepted, and the analytic methods employed should be meticulously documented and described.

The themes that underly these attributes are *credibility* and *accountability*. The link between a set of guidelines and the scientific evidence must be explicit, and scientific and clinical evidence should take precedence over expert judgment. Every set of guidelines should be accompanied by a clear statement of the strength of the relevant scientific evidence and expert judgment. When the empirical evidence has important limitations and experts reach conclusions that are not consistent with the evidence, then the rationale for departing from the evidence, such as it is, should be carefully explained. When expert judgment proceeds in the absence of direct empirical evidence about a particular clinical practice, as is often necessary, the general scientific reasoning and normative principles supporting the judgments should be described.

This report does not take a position on whether cost considerations should be explicitly factored into practice recommendations, although some committee members had strong views that they should be. However, documentation of projected health outcomes and costs to the degree possible is important to help developers and users of guidelines better understand the implications of following or not following the guidelines.

One of the committee's strongest recommendations is that the process of developing guidelines include participation by representatives of key affected groups and disciplines. Such participation increases the likelihood (1) that all relevant scientific evidence will be located and critically evaluated; (2) that practical problems with using the guidelines will be identified and addressed; and (3) that affected groups will see the guidelines as credible and will cooperate in implementing them. Participation by physicians, nurses, patients, and others can be achieved in several ways including membership on the development panel, testimony at public hearings, participation in focus groups, consultation during site visits, and provision of comments on draft guidelines.

The stringency of the attributes, especially taken together, is well recognized. Realistically, neither existing guidelines nor those likely to be developed by the agency in the foreseeable future will "score well" on all eight properties simultaneously. Indeed, near-perfect scores may always lie in the realm of aspiration rather than attainment. Moreover, the process of developing, assessing, using, evaluating, and revising guidelines will be evolutionary. There is today no proven "right way" to conduct this endeavor, even if there clearly are some "better ways." In addition, a balance needs to be maintained between an ideal process and one that is feasible. Guidelines that satisfactorily reflect the eight attributes proposed here may not be products of an ideal process, but in the committee's view they will be defensible.

RECOMMENDATIONS: IMPLEMENTATION AND EVALUATION

Although AHCPR and the Forum are responsible for implementing the government program for guidelines established in OBRA 89, the main work of implementing the guidelines themselves will be in the hands of physicians, nurses, health care administrators, and others. The agency, however, has important responsibilities for evaluating the impact of guidelines. The committee's discussions were limited by its charge and centered primarily on how the processes of implementation and evaluation can reinforce and extend the eight attributes of guidelines defined earlier.

One committee recommendation is that the agency instruct its expert panels and contractors to keep implementation and evaluation in mind as they develop guidelines. The tension between extraordinarily detailed or sophisticated guidelines and those that can be translated into usable medical review criteria or patient education materials must be recognized and dealt with during the development process, not after the fact.

Keeping implementation and evaluation in mind during guidelines development means, among other things, understanding the following.

• The credibility of the development process, the participants, and the scientific grounding of guidelines must be clear to intended users.

• A truly multidisciplinary approach to guidelines development will facilitate acceptance and use of guidelines by members of the groups represented and by other, secondary target groups.

• Guidelines should be specific, comprehensive, and flexible enough to be useful in the varied settings and circumstances of everyday medical practice and in the evolving programs to assess the appropriateness of care provided in these settings.

• Guidelines language, logic, and symbols should be easy to follow and unambiguous, so that movement from guidelines statements to educational tools, review criteria, or other instruments is unimpeded.

• The guidelines should specify what information about the clinical problem, the patient's circumstances and preferences, and the delivery setting should be recorded to permit later evaluation of the appropriateness of care (judged against criteria generated from the guidelines).

The implementation of guidelines is a diffuse, difficult-to-track process that will depend on many factors besides the quality and credibility of the guidelines. Among those factors are (1) the funding for dissemination and other implementation activities; (2) the supports and incentives for the guidelines to be used by physicians, nurses, health plans, and others; (3) the accessibility, scope, accuracy, and timeliness of a variety of intra- and interorganizational information systems; and (4) the ability of multiple parties to plan and execute the various steps needed to implement guidelines.

Users of guidelines will vary in their objectives and circumstances, and strategies for meeting particular user objectives will differ in their cost-effectiveness and manageability. Thus, different objectives and resources may call for different choices among the formats for guidelines (that is, their physical layout and logic), different roles for the available dissemination media, and different kinds of administrative supports for users of guidelines. Organizations with more resources (for example, libraries, video centers, telephone hotlines, personal computers, and network information systems) will be able to assist the use of guidelines in ways that are out of reach for less resource-rich organizations.

Medical review criteria and other evaluation instruments, if properly developed and sensitively applied, can create incentives for adherence to practice guidelines. If improperly developed and applied, they can undermine support for practice guidelines. Building on earlier IOM reports on utilization management and quality assurance, the committee discussed a few broad principles for the constructive use of medical review criteria and other evaluation tools derived from practice guidelines.

First, review criteria should be public with respect to their content and their development process. Second, when criteria are used to assess quality of care, deny payment for specific services, or take similar steps, an appeals process must be provided that is free from unreasonable complexity, delay, or other barriers. Third, review organizations should provide constructive information and feedback to physicians and other clinicians with the aim of improving practice rather than punishing missteps.

Fourth, review organizations should make their review activities as manageable and nonintrusive as possible. Such organizations contribute to the perceived and real "hassle factor" in medical care, which grows out of burgeoning demands by payers and others for more information on, and justification for, health services delivered or proposed. The Forum needs to be sensitive to this issue. It should also work with HCFA and other organizations to minimize negative effects from poor translation of otherwise good guidelines into review criteria, unduly stringent application of these criteria, or both.

The committee recognizes the critical importance of strong systems support for implementation. The complexities of creating such support within and across organizations are beyond the scope of this report but will be an important issue in further IOM work on practice guidelines.

With respect to the evaluation responsibilities of AHCPR and the Forum, the committee believes that the OBRA 89 provisions for evaluation are laudable but that the timetable is unrealistic. The Secretary of Health and Human Services is due to report on the impact of the first three guidelines by January 1, 1993. It is unlikely that measurable effects of these guidelines on the costs or quality of care will appear that quickly, and even if they do, it is unlikely that appropriate data on patient outcomes and program costs will be available and analyzed. Instead of a full-fledged evaluation, the agency can more reasonably be expected to provide a report on its evaluation plan, the steps being taken to implement the plan, and any preliminary evidence of impact.

DIVERSITY IN CLINICAL PRACTICES AND GUIDELINES

In its discussions, the committee repeatedly returned to questions of diversity in clinical practice and inconsistency among guidelines. Diversity in clinical practice can be acceptable or unacceptable. It may be reasonable when the scientific evidence to support different courses of care is uncertain. In addition, some degree of diversity may be warranted by differences in individual patient characteristics and preferences and variations in delivery system capacities related to locale, resources, and patient populations. However, even though practice variation based on scientific uncertainty or differences in values may be acceptable, both science and values are open to change. Thus, what is perceived as acceptable diversity in clinical practice may change over time.

Diversity in practice is unacceptable when it stems from poor practitioner skills, poor management of delivery systems, ignorance, or deliberate disregard of well-documented preferable practices. It should not be tolerated when it is a self-serving disguise for bad practices that harm people or waste scarce resources.

Guidelines can clarify what is acceptable and unacceptable variation in clinical practice, but that clarification itself has limits that may lead different groups to different and even inconsistent guidelines. Weak evidence is still weak evidence, although the processes described in Chapter 3 should allow the best use of whatever evidence is available. Nonetheless, these processes still leave room for differences of expert opinion about such issues as whether a flaw in research design "matters" or whether differences in results between two treatment alternatives are "clinically important" or only "statistically significant."

Inconsistency among guidelines can also arise from variations in values and tolerance for risk. People may simply differ in how they perceive different health outcomes and how they judge when benefits outweigh harms enough to make a service worth providing. One way to approach this kind of variation is to try to establish practitioner and patient attitudes toward different benefits and harms and then identify what is known about the probabilities of those different outcomes. In some cases, the developers of guidelines may take the further step of applying their own values, but others considering the guidelines later could look at the same information and perhaps come to different conclusions. Also, for some services and clinical conditions, the developers of guidelines may choose not to recommend a single course of action but to lay out alternative courses of treatment that may be appropriate depending on, for example, the preferences of a patient or the characteristics of a delivery setting or community.

In sum, merely identifying inconsistencies in guidelines says nothing about the legitimacy of those inconsistencies. Some inconsistencies may arise from biased or inept development processes. Some may result from reasonable differences in the interpretation of scientific evidence or in the application of patient, practitioner, or social values. Other inconsistencies may essentially disappear when the rationales for specific recommendations are closely examined. The challenge is to determine which explanation applies. Meticulous documentation of the evidence and rationales for guidelines will make this determination easier.

EXPECTATIONS FOR PRACTICE GUIDELINES

Today the field of guidelines development is a confusing mix of high expectations, competing organizations, conflicting philosophies, and ill-defined or incompatible objectives. It suffers from imperfect and incomplete scientific knowledge as well as imperfect and uneven means of applying that knowledge. Despite the good intentions of many involved parties, the enterprise lacks clearly articulated goals, coherent structures, and credible mechanisms for evaluating, improving, and coordinating guidelines development to meet social needs for good-quality, affordable health care.

This situation will not change overnight, even though many promising activities, including those sponsored by AHCPR, are under way. Thus, expectations of quick results should be restrained. Otherwise, dashed hopes may lead to calls for premature abandonment of a useful strategy for improving the appropriate use of health services and to the adoption of more draconian measures to control costs.[1]

The committee is also concerned about other expectations or assumptions that may be unrealistic. One such assumption is that guidelines development is a relatively simple or straightforward undertaking. It is not. For many clinical conditions and services, the science base is limited. Methods for analyzing evidence and developing expert opinions vary, but none of the rigorous methods can be properly applied by novices. Even in cases where considerable research has been done and sound methods

---

[1] In this vein, see the 1973 book by political scientists Jeffrey L. Pressman and Aaron B. Wildavsky, *Implementation: How Great Expectations in Washington Are Dashed in Oakland; Or, Why It's Amazing that Federal Programs Work at All, This Being a Saga of the Economic Development Administration as Told by Two Sympathetic Observers Who Seek to Build Morals on a Foundation of Ruined Hopes* (Berkeley, Calif.: University of California Press).

applied to analyze it, honest clinicians and analysts may still come to different conclusions from the same evidence. Agreement on facts may not be matched by agreement on what health benefits are desirable at which economic cost with what tolerable accompanying health risks.

Such conflicts about the interpretation of evidence and application of value judgments cannot be ignored. Indeed, the whole process of guidelines development has to be undertaken with great care at every stage: selecting participants, clarifying biases, adopting procedures and methods, identifying and analyzing evidence, considering alternatives, providing for independent reviews, preparing clear recommendations, and disclosing all important information about the process. Most of this report reinforces these points.

A second assumption of concern to the committee is that there is one right way to develop guidelines. There is not. Variations in the topics, the clinical disciplines involved, the purposes, and the audiences for guidelines will justify some differences in the specific methods for developing guidelines. However, to grant some methodological diversity is not to accept all approaches as equally good. Much remains to be tried and learned about the strengths and weaknesses of different methods.

A further questionable expectation, which is sometimes explicit but often unstated, is that practice guidelines will help control health care costs. They may not. The reasons for caution on this point are several. For instance, variation in practice does not, by itself, demonstrate that high-use patterns are necessarily the inappropriate ones. Moreover, even if high use can be identified as inappropriate, such identification does not automatically change behavior. An array of incentives for behavior change may be tried, but not all will succeed. Even if behavior changes, expenditures may not.

Some guidelines undoubtedly will save money by reducing the use of inappropriate services; some will increase costs by encouraging more use of underutilized services; and some will shift costs from one service or place or payer to another. The net impact on costs cannot be predicted with confidence, even if the priorities for guidelines development focus on clinical conditions for which overuse of expensive services is suspected. Nevertheless, if guidelines do succeed in improving the appropriateness and hence the *value* of this country's expenditures for medical care, then the endeavor will be a success.

This committee believes that AHCPR's practice guidelines effort has real potential to advance the state of the art in this field. The conditions for such success are demanding but not out of reach. In particular, expectations for the agency—and for practice guidelines per se—must be realistic regarding timetables and results. All parties concerned must act in good faith and keep the credibility and accountability of their actions in mind. Strict regard for the scientific rigor of the process is critical as is avoidance of premature closure on a single method of guidelines development.

Attention to implementation and evaluation needs to be factored into the development process at an early stage.

The Forum can underscore its intent to examine critically and improve its program and products in at least three ways. First, it should ask its expert panels for feedback on the strengths and weaknesses of the procedures followed. Second, it should pretest (or arrange for the pretesting of) all guidelines developed under its aegis. This can be done on a pilot basis in a real delivery setting, on a set of prototypical cases, or through both methods. Third, it should try to evaluate the effectiveness of intermediate actions (for example, formatting, dissemination, incentives) that are necessary if guidelines are to have their intended effects on health practices, outcomes, and costs. Each of these steps can be part of a learning process for the Forum and others.

NEXT STEPS FOR THE INSTITUTE OF MEDICINE

In May 1990, a new IOM committee began an 18-month study of the development, implementation, evaluation, and revision of clinical practice guidelines. Many of the issues raised in this report will be examined in depth during this second project, which is supported by the John A. Hartford Foundation, Inc., and the Public Health Service. In preparing its report and recommendations, the new committee will

- describe existing initiatives to develop, implement, and evaluate practice guidelines;
- identify the strengths and limitations of these efforts in light of the objectives and concerns of specific interest groups and society in general;
- describe different models of public and private action that might serve as prototypes for better structuring activities related to guidelines;
- analyze and assess the strengths, weaknesses, uncertainties, and trade-offs of different models in responding to identified problems and objectives; and
- propose a framework for better structuring the development, implementation, evaluation, and revision of practice guidelines.

In addition, the new committee will propose a practical methodology for AHCPR and others to employ in assessing guidelines before recommending or using them. It will focus on how the guidelines were developed, their scientific basis, their relevance to clinical practice, their clarity, and other characteristics. Such initial assessments will not substitute for later evaluations by government and others of the impact of a set of guidelines.

The committee's recommendations will cover both government and private activities, and its report will identify legislative, management, and other steps necessary to implement the recommendations. An active program of disseminating the committee's findings and recommendations is planned. The committee report should be released in the fall of 1991.

FINAL COMMENT

Fulfilling the mission and potential of the Forum will require heroic effort from a small staff, serious commitment from participants in the expert panels, and honest and practical support from the many involved and interested parties. Serious conceptual and practical issues remain to be confronted and resolved on a tight timetable with a modest budget. The undertaking will be strengthened if expectations are neither naively optimistic nor cynically pessimistic. This report suggests some of the ways in which the agency—with the help of many others *and* a stance of constructive realism—can move to meet its mandate.

1

Introduction and Background

. . .with [humility] comes not only a reverence for truth, but also a proper estimation of the difficulties encountered in our search for it.

William Osler, *Aequanimitas*

In November 1989, Congress amended the Public Health Service Act to create the Agency for Health Care Policy and Research (AHCPR). Under the terms of Public Law 101-239 (Appendix A), this agency has been given broad responsibilities for supporting research, data development, and other activities that will "enhance the quality, appropriateness, and effectiveness of health care services. . . ." The needs and priorities of the Medicare program are an important but not exclusive focus of the agency.

Many of AHCPR's responsibilities formerly belonged to the National Center for Health Services Research, which AHCPR has now replaced, but the emphasis on outcomes and effectiveness research is considerably stronger. Other functions of the agency are new, in particular, those involving a joint public-private enterprise to develop, disseminate, and evaluate guidelines for clinical practice under the sponsorship of the agency's Forum for Quality and Effectiveness in Health Care. (Appendix B provides some examples of guidelines already developed by public and private organizations.)

This report was prompted by AHCPR's request to the Institute of Medicine (IOM) for advice about how the agency and the Forum might approach their new and challenging responsibilities for practice guidelines.

19

The IOM agreed to appoint a study committee that would work quickly to provide technical assistance and advice on definition of terms, specification of key attributes of good guidelines, and certain aspects of planning for implementation and evaluation. This report largely confines itself to these specific and limited tasks.[1] It is not a how-to-do-it manual, a methodology text, a priority-setting exercise, or a primer on guidelines for those seeking an introduction to the subject. The report does, however, also aim to encourage more standardization and consistency in guidelines development, whether such development is supported directly by the Forum or is undertaken independently by medical societies and other organizations.

The committee believes that the AHCPR initiative, taken as a whole, has real potential to advance the state of the art for practice guidelines, strengthen the knowledge base for health care practice, and, hence, improve the appropriateness and effectiveness of health care. One objective of this report is to encourage realistic expectations about this potential by building a broader understanding of the difficult but important steps needed to move toward the goals for guidelines stated in P.L. 101-239, or, as it is often called, the Omnibus Budget Reconciliation Act of 1989 (OBRA 89).

CONTEXT

The legislation establishing AHCPR is one consequence of accumulated public and private frustration about the perceived health and economic consequences of inappropriate medical care. This frustration and the perceptions that give rise to it stem from many sources including ceaselessly escalating health care costs, wide variations in medical practice patterns, evidence that some health care services delivered in this country are of little or no value, and claims that various kinds of financial, educational, and organizational incentives can reduce inappropriate utilization (IOM, 1989).

The combination of high levels of expenditure and doubts about the value of that spending explains policymakers' interest in improving the scope and application of knowledge about what works and what does not work in medical care—and at what price. AHCPR is supporting an extensive agenda of outcomes and effectiveness research to add to the knowledge developed through other sources such as the randomized clinical trials funded by the National Institutes of Health. In fact, the major part of the agency's

---

[1] In addition, in May 1990, the IOM embarked on a new 18-month project funded by the John A. Hartford Foundation, Inc., and the Public Health Service to study both public and private activities to develop, use, and evaluate guidelines and to recommend a framework for better structuring of these activities where that is desirable and feasible (see Appendix C). The report of this study is planned for release in the fall of 1991.

work involves expanding the scope of knowledge rather than applying it. Of AHCPR's appropriation of nearly $100 million for fiscal year 1990, it planned to obligate around $2 million for the Forum's work on practice guidelines. (Some projects funded as research on outcomes will also involve the development of guidelines.) In any case, the agency's responsibilities for such guidelines reflect congressional recognition of the practical need for ways to translate knowledge into patient and practitioner decisions that improve the value received for the nation's health care spending.

More generally, the creation of a practice guidelines function within AHCPR can be seen as part of a significant cultural shift, a move away from unexamined reliance on professional judgment toward more structured support and accountability for such judgment (Physician Payment Review Commission, 1989; Roper et al., 1988). Reflecting one element of this shift, guidelines are intended to assist practitioners and patients in making health care decisions; reflecting the second aspect, they are to serve as a foundation for instruments to evaluate practitioner and health care system performance.

As the interest in practice guidelines has grown, so has scrutiny of existing guidelines and of processes for developing and using them (Brook, 1989; Eddy, 1987, 1988, 1990a–e, forthcoming (a,b); IOM, 1989, 1990; Leape, 1989, 1990; Physician Payment Review Commission, 1988a,b, 1989). This scrutiny leads to one clear conclusion: the systematic development, implementation, and evaluation of practice guidelines, based on rigorous clinical research and soundly generated professional consensus, have been progressing but also have serious limitations in method, scope, and substance. Concerns about these and other problems with practice guidelines contributed to the legislation creating AHCPR and the Forum.

OVERVIEW OF PRACTICE GUIDELINES INITIATIVES

Taken together, the public and private activities related to practice guidelines can be conceptualized, ideally, as having three basic stages: development, intervention, and evaluation. The second and third stages should—again, ideally—involve feedback loops to the first stage to prompt the revision of guidelines when omissions, technical obsolescence, or other problems are identified. Guidelines are thus dynamic, not static. They reflect the interplay of scientific and technological progress, real-world organizational pressures, and changes in social values.

To date, most government and other initiatives emphasize the first of the three stages, the development of practice guidelines. The intervention stage involves much more diffuse and less studied efforts to disseminate guidelines to target users and to encourage these users to actually apply the guidelines in making health care decisions. Only recently has much attention been paid to evaluating whether and why guidelines have any impact.

PUBLIC INITIATIVES

Under OBRA 89, AHCPR has responsibilities in several areas: (1) health services research including research on effectiveness, efficiency, and quality of health care with a particular emphasis on outcomes research; (2) development, collection, and dissemination of data; (3) health care technology assessment; and (4) practice guidelines. To promote activities in the area of practice guidelines, Congress created a unit within AHCPR, the Office of the Forum for Quality and Effectiveness in Health Care. As described in more detail later in this chapter, the Forum must "arrange for" the development and periodic review and updating of

> (1) clinically relevant guidelines that may be used by physicians, educators, and health care practitioners to assist in determining how diseases, disorders, and other health conditions can most effectively and appropriately be prevented, diagnosed, treated, and managed clinically; and
> (2) standards of quality, performance measures, and medical review criteria through which health care providers and other appropriate entities may assess or review the provision of health care and assure the quality of such care.

As explained by one individual intimately involved in the development of this legislation, the phrase *arrange for* is one key indicator of the "extent to which the legislation was structured to create a public-private enterprise with respect to guideline development. The Forum develops no guidelines; guidelines are not to be federal creations" (Peter Budetti, George Washington University, personal communication, July 13, 1989). The committee suspects, nonetheless, that most people will continue to use the term *develop* to describe what the Forum does in this area.

Other agencies of the federal government have or have recently had responsibilities related to practice guidelines. These agencies include the National Institutes of Health, the U.S. Preventive Services Task Force,[2] and the Health Care Financing Administration (HCFA) and its contracting carriers, fiscal intermediaries, and peer review organizations. HCFA and its contractors have developed criteria for reviewing services provided to Medicare beneficiaries. These criteria and their application, neither of which are examined here, have been criticized for lack of rigor and accountability (Institute of Medicine, 1990; Physician Payment Review Commission, 1988a, 1989).

---

[2] The *Guide to Clinical Preventive Services* prepared by the U.S. Preventive Services Task Force (1989) is a useful text to read in conjunction with this report, although this report is not specifically cross-referenced to the guide.

PRIVATE INITIATIVES

Guidelines for clinical practice, broadly defined, are not new. The processes of organized clinical education require various sorts of guidelines as do the processes of professional licensure, board certification, quality assurance, utilization review, and other aspects of health services administration. However, in recent years, the interest in practice guidelines of the medical community and others has grown exponentially.

The level of interest in guidelines is not all that has changed. Today, there is a much greater emphasis on formal procedures and methods for arriving at a more widely scrutinized and endorsed consensus about what is appropriate clinical practice.

Among the medical groups involved for some years with the development of guidelines are the American Academy of Family Physicians, the American College of Cardiology, the American College of Physicians, and the American Society of Anesthesiologists. In the research community, the RAND Corporation has pioneered the development of important tools and strategies. Newer initiatives are being undertaken or planned by the American Board of Medical Specialties, the American Medical Association, the Council of Medical Specialty Societies, and the academic medical and health services research community.

Insurers, health maintenance organizations (HMOs), utilization management firms, and similar organizations have not ignored the potential of practice guidelines as a basis for refusing payment for inappropriate care. For example, several years ago the Blue Cross and Blue Shield Association began its Medical Necessity Project, which supported and cooperated with researchers and some medical organizations in their efforts to identify obsolete procedures and set guidelines for the appropriate use of many diagnostic and treatment services. The Health Insurance Association of America recently established a similar function, and the Group Health Association of America has been sponsoring programs on guidelines development. Furthermore, individual members of each of these associations are involved in additional efforts to develop or adapt practice guidelines to meet the needs of their different health plans. In addition, the activities of dozens of firms supplying utilization management services to health plan sponsors have focused attention on the quality, scope, and accessibility of the criteria they use to review care on a prospective or concurrent basis.

The guidelines development efforts of private organizations are thus proceeding on many fronts. Some coordinating strategies are emerging, but important problems remain—unexplained conflicts among guidelines, neglected topics, lack of follow-up, and incomplete public disclosure of the evidence, participants, and methods used to develop sets of guidelines. There is no independent entity to certify that guidelines are sound in

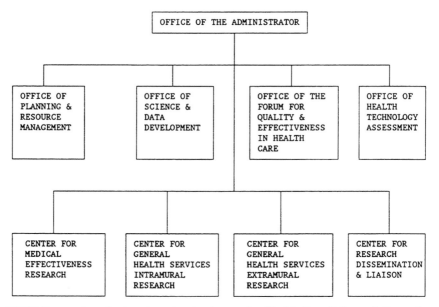

FIGURE 1-1   Organization chart for the Agency for Health Care Policy and Research. SOURCE: Office of the Forum for Quality and Effectiveness in Health Care.

method and content and no "national bureau of standards" to set standards for methods of guidelines development or their content. The legislation creating AHCPR is one response to some of these problems.

SPECIFIC RESPONSIBILITIES OF AHCPR

The legislative mandate for AHCPR and its Forum sets forth several specific responsibilities; it also identifies priorities and establishes certain procedural requirements. In planning to implement this mandate, the Forum has consulted with a broad array of interested individuals and organizations. The IOM committee is itself part of this consultation process. Other efforts include presentations, meetings, and mailings to medical societies, health care organizations, and other individuals and groups.

The following discussion notes the main elements of the legislative mandate and describes the agency's initial steps to fulfill its responsibilities. Figure 1-1 is an organization chart for the agency.

DEADLINES AND PRIORITIES

By January 1, 1991, AHCPR—acting through the Forum—must arrange for the development of an initial set of guidelines, standards, performance measures, and review criteria for at least three clinical treatments or conditions. AHCPR is also responsible for seeing that the guidelines developed under its auspices are updated.

OBRA 89 created the Advisory Council for Health Care Policy, Research, and Evaluation to advise the Secretary of the Department of Health and Human Services (DHHS) and the administrator of AHCPR on priorities and strategy. It also established the Subcouncil on Outcomes and Guidelines (of the Advisory Council) to provide advice on priorities and strategy for guidelines development and outcomes research.

A key explicit objective of the guidelines legislation is to help improve the quality, appropriateness, and effectiveness of health care. More implicit—yet widely recognized—is the hope that guidelines will help control health care costs. In selecting conditions for guidelines development, the agency is to consider the extent to which guidelines for the condition can be expected to reduce variations in health care services and outcomes and to improve care for significant numbers of people.

Priorities for the initial sets of guidelines to be developed by January 1, 1991, are more specific and stipulate that the clinical conditions involved (1) account for significant expenditures in Medicare, (2) show significant variation in the frequency or type of treatment provided, or (3) otherwise meet the needs and priorities of the Medicare program. Target users for the guidelines, standards, review criteria, and performance measures are "physicians, health care practitioners, medical educators, medical review organizations, and consumers."

At this writing, the Forum is considering initial guidelines development activities in the following areas:

- Cataract surgery
- Benign prostatic hyperplasia
- Clinical depression
- Sickle-cell disease
- Management of incontinence
- Management of chronic pain
- Management of skin integrity and decubitus ulcers
- Ambulatory care for human immunodeficiency virus infection

All of these areas except ambulatory care for patients with human immunodeficiency virus had panel chairs appointed as of July 1, 1990. These areas cover a wide variety of patients (not exclusively the elderly) and are relevant for a variety of practitioners including physicians, nurses, nurse practitioners, and social workers. According to Forum Director Stephen King, these conditions and treatments are being considered because they are important health problems characterized by a state of clinical knowledge and professional judgment that warrants a guidelines development effort and for which guidelines can be expected to reduce inappropriate variation in services, improve the quality of care, and produce better health outcomes. Additional clinical conditions or treatments will be identified on an ongoing basis. The Forum expects to have several sets of guidelines under development or assessment at any given time.

DEVELOPMENT PROCEDURES AND REQUIREMENTS

The director of the Forum may contract with public and nonprofit private organizations to develop and update guidelines. The director may also convene expert panels that can either develop guidelines or review guidelines developed by contractors. (There is some disagreement about whether the legislation requires the director to use both the contracting and the panel mechanisms.) The process must include appropriate consultations with interested individuals and organizations, including general and specialty medical organizations and physicians in a variety of practice settings. In addition, the director of the Forum must establish the standards for methods and procedures to be followed by the contractors and expert panels. The legislation permits pilot-testing of the guidelines.

One difficult task for the Forum has been deciding whether to convene expert panels to develop guidelines or to contract with outside entities. Initially, the Forum has adopted the first approach, namely, the convening of its own expert panels. As the guidelines program expands, the Forum may—some say, must—use the contracting mechanism. Forum staff are discussing such arrangements with a number of organizations.

In addition to arranging for the development of guidelines by expert panels or contractors, the agency may adopt guidelines developed independently of the Forum if they meet the requirements established by the legislation. As described by one person involved in the drafting of OBRA 89, "This is a critical addition to the current ad hoc system. For the first time, interested parties could turn over their products to a publicly constituted, disinterested body for scrutiny. After appropriate modification, the original guidelines would achieve an imprimatur of sorts from the disinterested body" (Peter Budetti, George Washington University, personal communication, July 13, 1990).

DISSEMINATION

The responsibilities of the Forum extend beyond the development of guidelines to their dissemination. The legislation specifies that the director of the Forum shall promote the dissemination of guidelines through organizations representing health care providers and health care consumers, peer review organizations, accrediting bodies, and other appropriate entities. In addition, the guidelines must be presented in formats appropriate for use by practitioners, medical educators, and medical care reviewers. Among the first steps the agency is taking to promote the dissemination of guidelines is to work with the National Library of Medicine for inclusion of the guidelines in the library's various information systems.

USE OF GUIDELINES

The legislation establishing AHCPR and the Forum states that the Secretary of Health and Human Services "shall provide for the use of the [initial sets of] guidelines. . .to improve the quality, effectiveness, and appropriateness of care" provided under the Medicare program. No further details are offered. Presumably, providing for the use of the guidelines will require that HCFA and its contracting fiscal intermediaries, carriers, and peer review organizations take steps to incorporate medical review criteria and other evaluation instruments into their programs to review care provided to Medicare beneficiaries. Discussion of these matters is at the most preliminary stages within DHHS.

EVALUATION AND FURTHER RESEARCH

The Secretary of Health and Human Services must determine the impact of the initial set of guidelines on the cost, quality, appropriateness, and effectiveness of health care and report these findings to Congress by January 1, 1993. Because an adequate evaluation within this time period is virtually impossible (see Chapter 4), the agency expects to provide Congress with a status report at the start of 1993 rather than a complete evaluation. More generally, the director of the Forum is to conduct and support evaluations of the impact of guidelines on clinical practice. In addition, the director is to recommend research projects to the AHCPR administrator that are related to (1) evaluating outcomes of health care services and procedures, (2) developing standards and criteria for the guidelines development process (what are called "attributes" in this report), and (3) promoting the use of the guidelines, standards, performance measures, and review criteria developed under the Forum's auspices.

THE INSTITUTE OF MEDICINE COMMITTEE AND PROJECT

To conduct the study requested by AHCPR, the IOM appointed a committee of experts in January 1990 (Appendix D). Members were selected on the basis of their expertise and familiarity with characteristics and uses of medical practice guidelines, desirable properties or attributes of guidelines, and technical methods for preparing them. The committee included practicing physicians, individuals experienced in the development of guidelines, current and potential users of guidelines, and representatives of relevant other disciplines such as nursing, law, and economics.

The IOM organized and conducted two meetings of the committee, one in February and the other in April 1990. A major immediate goal of the group was to help the Forum prepare to award and administer contracts for the development of guidelines for three clinical treatments or conditions. IOM staff provided background materials for the study committee that included a survey of guidelines activity (Audet and Greenfield, 1989), a case study of the mammography screening guideline for women aged 40 to 49 (Field, 1989), a chapter on attributes of quality of care indicators from an earlier IOM report (IOM, 1990), selected journal articles, reports from the American Medical Association and other medical organizations, and two volumes of examples of guidelines and formats from various sources. The committee also received status reports from the Forum director at each meeting. The April meeting included presentations by Mark Chassin and Sheldon Greenfield on practical implementation and evaluation issues. Chapters 2, 3, and 4 describe sources of information in more detail. In addition, IOM staff prepared papers for review by the committee as a basis for recommendations and the final report.

Staff from the Forum attended both meetings and received copies of all draft and background materials prepared for the committee. After each meeting, IOM staff prepared meeting summaries and circulated them to committee members for their review and comment. Based on committee discussion of staff papers and the meeting summaries, this report was drafted, circulated to the committee for comment, revised, and then submitted for review in accordance with IOM and National Research Council report review policies. After revisions were made based on the latter review, this document was produced, constituting the committee's final report.

OVERVIEW OF THE REPORT

The next chapter discusses definitions of key terms—why the definitions are needed, how the committee approached this task, and what the literature says about terminology. It sets forth specific definitions for practice guidelines, medical review criteria, and standards of quality, and a provisional definition for performance measures.

Chapter 3 takes up the attributes of good guidelines. It again describes how the committee approached the topic and what the literature says about desirable properties of guidelines. The themes that underlie this discussion are the importance of credibility and full disclosure of the processes, sources, methods, and participants in guidelines development. The committee has identified eight attributes of guidelines: validity, reliability/ reproducibility, clinical applicability, clinical flexibility, clarity, multidisciplinary process, scheduled review, and documentation. The stringency of these attributes, especially taken together, is well recognized, and the committee realizes that a balance needs to be maintained between an ideal process and a feasible one. In a second IOM project on practice guidelines (Appendix C), one task will be to take the conceptual attributes described in Chapter 3 and develop an operationally useful instrument for assessing how specific sets of guidelines conform to these attributes.

In Chapter 4, the committee concentrates on implementation and evaluation. This chapter differentiates between the implementation of a government program for guidelines (which includes hiring staff and convening expert panels) and the implementation or application of guidelines after they are developed. It also differentiates between evaluating the impact of clinical practices and evaluating the impact of practice guidelines.

Chapter 5 summarizes the committee's recommendations and conclusions. The recommendations, although sensitive to broader congressional expectations for the new agency, reflect the committee's relatively limited charge to advise the Public Health Service on definitions and attributes of guidelines.

CONCLUSIONS AND CAUTIONARY NOTES

Today, the field of guidelines development is a confusing mix of high expectations, competing organizations, conflicting philosophies, and ill-defined or incompatible objectives. It suffers from imperfect and incomplete scientific knowledge as well as imperfect and uneven means of applying that knowledge. Despite the good intentions of many of the parties involved, the enterprise lacks coherent structures and credible mechanisms for evaluating, improving, and coordinating guidelines development to meet society's needs for good-quality, affordable health care.

This situation will not change overnight, even though many promising activities, including those sponsored by AHCPR, are under way. Consequently, expectations for quick results should be somewhat restrained. Otherwise, dashed hopes may lead to calls for premature abandonment of a useful strategy for improving the appropriate use of health care services and to the adoption of more draconian measures to control costs.

The committee is also concerned about other unrealistic expectations or assumptions—for example, the assumption that guidelines development is a relatively simple or straightforward undertaking. It is not. For many clinical conditions and services, the scientific base is limited. (This is one reason why it is important that the guidelines and knowledge development functions of AHCPR be coordinated.) Methods for analyzing evidence and developing expert opinion vary, but none of the rigorous methods can be properly applied by novices. Where considerable research has been done and good methods have been applied to analyze it, honest clinicians and analysts may come to different conclusions using the same evidence. Agreement on facts may not be accompanied by agreement on what health benefits are desirable at which economic cost with what tolerable accompanying health risks.

Such conflicts about the interpretation of evidence and the application of value judgments cannot be ignored. Indeed, the whole process of guidelines development must be undertaken with care at every stage: selecting participants, clarifying biases, adopting procedures and methods, identifying and analyzing evidence, considering alternatives, providing for independent reviews, preparing clear recommendations, and disclosing all important information about the process. This report is intended to reinforce these points.

A second assumption of concern to the committee is that there is only one right way to develop guidelines. There is not. Variations in the topics, the clinical disciplines involved, the purposes, and the audiences for guidelines will justify some differences in specific development methods. However, to grant some methodological diversity is not to accept all approaches as equally good. Chapter 3 pursues this point but notes that much remains to be tried and learned about the strengths and weaknesses of different guidelines development methods.

One further questionable expectation, which is sometimes explicit but often unstated, is that practice guidelines will help control health care costs.[3] They may not. The reasons for caution on this point are several. For instance, variation in practice does not, by itself, demonstrate that the high-use patterns are the inappropriate ones. Moreover, even if high use can be identified as inappropriate, such identification does not automatically change behavior. An array of incentives for behavioral change may be tried, but not all will succeed. Even if behavior changes, expenditures may

---

[3] See, for example, the discussions of expenditure targets, volume performance standards, and guidelines in the Physician Payment Review Commission's 1989 (Chapters 11 and 12) and 1990 (Chapter 2) reports.

not. Some guidelines undoubtedly will save money by reducing the use of inappropriate services; some will increase costs by encouraging more use of underutilized services; and some will shift costs from one service, place, or payer to another. The net impact on costs cannot be predicted with confidence, even if the priorities for guidelines development focus on clinical conditions for which overuse of expensive services is suspected.

One of the main areas of disagreement among committee members involved precisely how costs should be considered in the development of practice guidelines. Some committee members believed that all guidelines should incorporate judgments about cost-effectiveness whereas the majority called for the development process, at a minimum, to include projections of cost effects. In any case, if guidelines do succeed in improving the value of the nation's expenditures of medical care by allowing more informed individual and social decisionmaking that in turn shifts expenditures from less to more appropriate forms of care, then the endeavor will be successful.

As stated at the outset of this chapter, the committee believes that AHCPR has the potential to strengthen the knowledge base for health care decisionmaking and contribute to the development of practice guidelines. It can be an important element in the much broader array of public and private actions to improve the quality and effectiveness of health care. This report suggests some ways in which the agency—with the help of many others and a stance of constructive realism—can move to meet its mandate.

REFERENCES

Audet, A., and Greenfield, S. A Survey of Current Activities in Practice Guideline Development. Paper prepared for an IOM Meeting on Medical Practice Guidelines: Looking Ahead, November 8, 1989, Washington, D.C.

Brook, R. Practice Guidelines and Practicing Medicine. Are They Compatible? *Journal of the American Medical Association* 262:3027–3030, 1989.

Eddy, D. Clinical Policies. Pp. 47–54 in *Proceedings. Standards of Quality in Patient Care: The Importance and Risks of Standard Setting.* Invitational Conference, Council of Medical Specialty Societies, Washington, D.C., September 1987.

Eddy, D. Methods for Designing Guidelines. Paper prepared for the Physician Payment Review Commission. Duke University, Durham, N.C., 1988.

Eddy, D. Comparing Benefits and Harms: The Balance Sheet. *Journal of the American Medical Association* 263:2493–2505, 1990a.

Eddy, D. Guidelines for Policy Statements: The Explicit Approach. *Journal of the American Medical Association* 263:2239–2240, 1990b.

Eddy, D. Practice Policies—Guidelines for Methods. *Journal of the American Medical Association* 263:1839–1841, 1990c.

Eddy, D. Practice Policies—What are They? *Journal of the American Medical Association* 263:877–880, 1990d.

Eddy, D. Practice Policies—Where Do They Come From? *Journal of the American Medical Association* 263:1265–1275, 1990e.

Eddy, D. Designing a Practice Policy: Standards, Guidelines, and Options. *Journal of the American Medical Association*, forthcoming (a).

Eddy, D. *A Manual for Assessing Health Practices and Designing Practice Policies* (draft dated May 31, 1989). American College of Physicians, forthcoming (b).

Field, M. Health Policy and Medical Practice Guidelines: The Case of Mammography Screening for Women Under 50. Paper prepared for an IOM Meeting on Medical Practice Guidelines: Looking Ahead, November 8, 1989, Washington, D.C.

Institute of Medicine. *Controlling Costs and Changing Patient Care? The Role of Utilization Management*, B. Gray and M. Field, eds. Washington, D.C.: National Academy Press, 1989.

Institute of Medicine. *Medicare: A Strategy for Quality Assurance*, vols. 1 and 2, K. Lohr, ed. Washington, D.C.: National Academy Press, 1990.

Leape, L. Unnecessary Surgery. *Health Services Research* 24:352–407, 1989.

Leape, L. Practice Guidelines and Standards: An Overview. *Quality Review Bulletin* 16:42–49, 1990.

Physician Payment Review Commission. *Annual Report to Congress*. Washington, D.C., 1988a.

Physician Payment Review Commission. Improving the Quality of Care: Clinical Research and Practice Guidelines. Appendix I. Background Paper for the Conference on Practice Guidelines, Washington, D.C., October 1988b.

Physician Payment Review Commission. *Annual Report to Congress*. Washington, D.C., 1989.

Physician Payment Review Commission. *Annual Report to Congress*. Washington, D.C., 1990.

Roper, W., Winkenwerder, W., Hackbarth, G., et al. Effectiveness in Health Care. An Initiative to Evaluate and Improve Medical Practice. *New England Journal of Medicine* 319:1197–1202, 1988.

U.S. Preventive Services Task Force. *Guide to Clinical Preventive Services: An Assessment of the Effectiveness of 169 Interventions*. Baltimore, Md.: Williams & Wilkins, 1989.

2

Definitions of Key Terms

"When I use a word," Humpty Dumpty said, in rather a scornful tone, "it means just what I choose it to mean—neither more nor less."

"The question is," said Alice, "whether you *can* make words mean so many different things."

"The question is," said Humpty Dumpty, "which is to be master—that's all."

Lewis Carroll, *Through the Looking Glass*

If AHCPR and the Forum are to proceed confidently with their mission, they need clear, broadly acceptable definitions of four key terms, which were used in the legislation establishing the agency: (1) practice guidelines, (2) medical review criteria, (3) standards of quality, and (4) performance measures. Neither the final legislation nor preceding House or Senate bills offered definitions of these concepts.

The four key terms employed in OBRA 89 have been defined and used in quite disparate ways. Words like *guidelines* and *standards* may mean one thing to clinicians, another to purchasers, and yet another to attorneys. (The study directors for this project discovered early in their work that they were using these terms differently.) Moreover, the same person may use the same term differently in different contexts. Table 2-1 suggests how context influences usage and terminology.

Further complicating the semantic and conceptual situation are other frequently used terms that are not mentioned in the legislation—terms

TABLE 2-1 Influence of Context on Terminology

Context	Influence
Users	Users may be practitioners, payers, or consumers. Common practitioner terms include "practice guidelines" and "algorithms." Consumer terms include "patient information" (such as "postoperative instructions"). For insurers, terms such as "medical necessity" and "standard practice" are used in discussions of health plan coverage, and lawyers refer to "community standards" in malpractice cases.
Purposes	Purposes may include practice management, practitioner or patient education, quality assessment, and payment determination. Purposes and users overlap to some extent, but even a single user such as a clinician may talk at one time about "protocols" or "indications" for an intervention and at another time about "clinical indicators" or "occurrence screens" to flag potential problems for further review in quality assurance programs.
Timing	Prospective, concurrent, or retrospective uses may require very different formulations. Practice management guidelines are intended to guide care prospectively, and "precertification criteria" are used to review proposed care on a case-by-case basis. Continued stay review has employed "length of stay norms." Retrospective review may use "screens" and analyses of practice patterns.
Consensus	A number of terminological distinctions have been based on the strength of scientific evidence or expert consensus about what is effective or ineffective medical care. One formulation uses "standard," "guideline," and "option" to indicate decreasing levels of information about the likely outcomes of an intervention and decreasing levels of consensus about preferences for different outcomes. Other frameworks use gradations such as class I, II, and III to indicate conditions for which the application is justified, for which there is divergent opinion, and for which it is unjustified. Still other classifications use such terms as "appropriate," "equivocal," and "inappropriate."
Complexity	At one extreme are "rules of thumb" and "dicta," which are often stated very tersely. At the other extreme lie detailed algorithms, decision trees, and "criteria maps."

such as *clinical indicators*, *practice parameters*, *norms*, and *practice policies* (Meyer, 1989). Some people may treat certain of these terms as synonymous; others may make strong conceptual or practical distinctions. Given this abundance of terminology and meaning, it is helpful to recall what Donabedian (1981:409) said when discussing norms, criteria, and standards: "we have used these words in so many different ways that we no longer clearly understand each other when we say them. But we. . .do not have the liberty of abandoning them. . . . Our more reasonable course. . .

is to see whether we can clarify the existing nomenclature, barnacled and misshapen though it may be with the encrustation of careless past usage."

Guided by the spirit of this observation, the committee's objectives are limited: to provide definitions that are clear, realistic, and practical for use with expert panels, contractors, and others. These definitions are not expected to serve all users for all purposes; however, they should permit clear communication between the Forum and the many organizations and interests with which it must work.

THE COMMITTEE'S APPROACH

The committee began its definitional exercise by consulting the literature on practice guidelines, quality of care, and related topics. This body of work contains a number of thoughtful efforts by practitioners, researchers, policy analysts, and others to define and explain key terms. In addition, the committee used standard English and American dictionaries, which provided common uses of the four terms. Congressional and agency staff were also consulted.

In proposing definitions, the committee wanted to make its rationale and purposes explicit. To that end, it identified six desirable, although not fully compatible, characteristics of a definition.

1. Each definition should be *parsimonious*; that is, it should include the minimum necessary distinguishing characteristics of the concept in question. It should exclude elements that are not essential to make the definition clear and useful (for example, priorities for action, contingencies, or desired characteristics for "good" instances of the concept).

2. Each definition should be *consistent with customary social and professional usage*, insofar as reasonable given other objectives.

3. Each definition should be *consistent with legislative language*, insofar as reasonable.

4. Each definition should be *practically and symbolically acceptable* to important interests, insofar as reasonable.

5. Each definition should *not be easily misunderstood or misused*, insofar as reasonable.

6. A word or phrase should *not be defined in terms of itself* (for example, a practice guideline should not be defined using words such as "guiding medical practice"); the definition should *not be tautological*.

With these criteria in mind, the committee reviewed definitions in common and professional use, developed draft definitions of terms, and then revised the definitions based on committee discussion. The following sections of the chapter describe the results of this process for each of the four key terms.

PRACTICE GUIDELINES

The committee began by defining the term *guidelines* because it appears to be the term most commonly and comprehensively used in professional and policy discussions. It is employed in this general way in the legislation establishing AHCPR.

COMMON USAGE: THE DICTIONARY

The *Random House Dictionary of the English Language* (1987) dates the American origin of *guideline* to 1775–1785, presumably in its literal usage as a "rope or cord that serves to guide one's steps especially over rocky terrain, through underground passages, etc." Its more metaphorical use— "any guide or indication of a future course of action"—is a recent addition. The verb "to guide" is given several meanings including "to supply with advice or counsel." This dictionary notes that the term "implies continuous presence or agency in showing or indicating a course" as distinct from pilot, steer, escort, direct, or lead.

The *Compact Edition of the Oxford English Dictionary (OED)* (1971) does not define *guideline* directly but includes it in a set of examples of attributes of technical appliances and machinery parts (e.g., guideline for a saw). It defines the verb "to guide" in much the same way as above: to direct the course of (a physical action, for instance) and to lead in a course of action or the direction of events.

PROFESSIONAL AND TECHNICAL USAGE

American Medical Association (AMA) (J. Kelly, director of the Office of Quality Assurance, letter dated April 26, 1990): "Guideline: Recommendation for patient management which identifies a particular management strategy or a range of management strategies. Practice parameters: Strategies for patient management developed to assist physicians in clinical decision-making."

The Forum (S. King, Forum director, personal communication, January 1990): "A guideline is a description of the process of care which will permit health to improve, and which has the potential of improving the quality of medical decision-making" (provisional definition).

U.S. General Accounting Office (G. Silberman, assistant director, Program Evaluation and Methodology Division, letter dated October 16, 1989, to medical specialty societies): "[G]uidance—by whatever name—that aids practicing physicians and others in the medical community (and consumers, if included) in day-to-day decisions by describing the degree of appropriateness and the relative effectiveness of alternate approaches to detecting,

THE COMMITTEE'S DEFINITION: PRACTICE GUIDELINE

Practice guidelines are systematically developed statements to assist practitioner and patient decisions about appropriate health care for specific clinical circumstances.

Practice guidelines assist patients and practitioners in making decisions about health care. To that end, they describe clearly appropriate care, clearly inappropriate care, or care about which the scientific evidence and consensus are equivocal. Guidelines focus on specific clinical circumstances, which may sometimes include clinically relevant organizational factors, community characteristics, social variables, and similar influences on health care delivery.[1] They should be developed in a formal, systematic way that is fully documented, as discussed in Chapter 3 of this report.

As defined here, practice guidelines include such varied means of assisting clinical decisionmaking as pathway guidelines or practice algorithms, boundary guidelines or appropriateness criteria, and practice parameters. (Appendix B contains examples of different styles of guidelines.) The choice of approach in developing guidelines will depend on their purpose, the intended users and sites of care, and the clarity and quality of the scientific evidence on which they are based.

Judged in terms of the principles the committee set forth for good definitions, this definition is reasonably succinct, generally consistent with common, professional, and legislative usage, and not tautological. The element of advice or counsel in the committee definition differentiates *guideline* from such terms as *suggestion* (which is weaker than advice or counsel), *information* (which is less goal oriented), and *criterion* (which, as discussed below, adds the element of evaluation). The definition goes beyond the dictionary by adding the requirement that the advice or counsel be "systematically developed." This element is mentioned by many health care researchers and medical organizations either explicitly or implicitly through such phrases as "formal development" and "well understood" and references to the scientific literature.

Based on its discussions in meetings and in other quarters, the committee believes its definition of practice guideline is, for the most part, practically and symbolically acceptable to varied groups. When combined with the other definitions offered here and the specification of desirable attributes of guidelines, the definition should be as little subject to misuse and misunderstanding as is possible, given the semantic diversity described

---

[1] Clinically relevant organizational factors include the equipment, facilities, personnel, and skill levels available within a particular health care institution or local community. Clinically relevant social factors include the patient's home and family circumstances.

earlier. A few areas of potential controversy can be anticipated, however, and they are discussed below.

Guidelines and the Strength of Evidence

In and of itself, the committee's definition of practice guidelines does not explicitly require that guidelines describe the strength of the scientific evidence or consensus associated with a set of guidelines. Rather than being part of the definition, the committee views this property as an attribute that good guidelines must have (see Chapter 3). Every set of guidelines developed or adopted by the Forum should be accompanied by clear statements about their strength, and the evidence for such statements should be cited. When the evidence is extremely strong and professional judgment is virtually unanimous, the guideline may be treated as a standard of practice permitting few if any exceptions. When the evidence is equivocal, the guideline may only identify currently acceptable practice options.[2]

This use of the phrases *standard of practice* and *practice option* is consistent with Eddy's usage as described earlier. However, the committee's use of the term *guideline* is equivalent to Eddy's umbrella use of the phrase *practice policy*. The committee's primary reason for using *guideline* as the general label was that the term is used this way in the legislation establishing AHCPR and by other sources such as the Physician Payment Review Commission. Admittedly, the committee risks creating some confusion by using the phrase *standard of practice*, given the OBRA 89 reference to "standards of quality," but it judges that the risk is acceptable because the term is useful and, indeed, hard to avoid.

Relation of Guidelines to Review Criteria and Other Evaluation Tools

In the committee's reading, OBRA 89 does not use the terms *standards of quality*, *performance measures*, and *medical review criteria* as synonyms for *practice guidelines*. Instead, it links these three terms to evaluating practice rather than to assisting practitioners and patients.[3] Although the Forum is required to arrange for the development of these tools, other sponsors of guidelines may do no more than offer general observations on how the guidelines should or should not be used in evaluating practitioner decisions and outcomes. For various practical or technical reasons, some elements

---

[2] Some health care organizations or health benefit plans may rule out certain of these options given their objectives, resource limits, or other constraints (Havighurst, forthcoming). Such decisions, however, are distinct from scientifically and professionally based judgments about practices that are acceptable options for clinicians.

[3] See sections 912(a)(1) and (a)(2) of Title IX of the Public Health Service Act as amended by P.L. 101-239.

of a set of guidelines may have no corresponding review criteria or other practice evaluation tools at all.

For example, one guideline of the U.S. Preventive Services Task Force (1989:108) states that "screening for congenital hypothyroidism is recommended for all neonates during the first week of life." This statement and a subsequent one defining specific tests to be used could be directly translated into a criterion for reviewing care for a specific neonatal case or for reviewing the pattern of neonatal care provided by a practitioner or an institution. In contrast, the further statement by the Task Force that "*it may be prudent* to perform regular physical examinations of the thyroid in persons with a history of upper-body irradiation" (emphasis added) would be difficult to translate into a criterion for assessing either case-by-case or aggregate performance. Of course, even though certain statements about neonates *could* be used for medical review performance, determining that they *should* be so used requires a decision that the benefits of such a review in improving health or other desired outcomes warrant the administrative steps and costs that a review would entail.

To cite a different example with respect to screening for hearing loss, the Preventive Services Task Force (1989:198), recommends that "screening of workers for noise-induced hearing loss should be performed in the context of existing worksite programs and occupational medicine guidelines." Such a statement may have some value for patients or clinicians without itself generating a review criterion in the context considered in this report.

Definition of Appropriate Care

Because the concept of *appropriate* care or appropriateness is crucial to the committee's definition of practice guidelines and is itself the subject of some differences and confusion in usage, the committee considered it necessary to explicitly define this concept. Brook and his colleagues at the RAND Corporation define appropriate care as follows: when "the expected health benefit [exceeds] the expected negative consequences. . .by a sufficiently wide margin that the procedure [is] worth doing" (see, e.g., Park et al., 1986:6). Conversely, care is inappropriate when the expected harms exceed the expected health benefits.[4]

Care may range from clearly appropriate to clearly inappropriate. Care that is not described by scientific evidence and expert judgment as either clearly one or the other may be termed equivocal. A practice might be

---

[4]Health benefits include increased life expectancy, better functional status, and reduced morbidity, pain, and anxiety. Negative health outcomes are the opposites of these qualities. Both short-term and long-term positive and negative outcomes should be examined to determine appropriateness.

labeled equivocal for empirical reasons; that is, the benefits and harms are uncertain. It might also be described as equivocal because of ambivalence, for instance, when the benefits are known to exceed harms but to such a trivial or small degree that raters are reluctant to call the practice appropriate. In this latter case, value judgments may have much to do with whether a practice is considered "worth" providing (or receiving), and these judgments may rest on considerations of cost and other matters.

Guidelines and Costs

The committee's definition of appropriate care does not require that guidelines be based on judgments about the cost-effectiveness of particular clinical practices; neither does it preclude it. As discussed in Chapter 3, the committee concludes that, insofar as feasible, developers of guidelines should consider costs and should include information with the guidelines that allows others to make their own cost-benefit or cost-effectiveness judgments. The committee's decision not to incorporate an explicit reference to costs in the definition of practice guidelines or appropriate care reflects a value judgment that was not shared by all committee members. The majority, however, believed that the emphasis on clinical decisionmaking should be paramount.

In addition, some committee members strongly disagreed with the committee's decision not to refer explicitly to third-party payers and others in the definition of practice guidelines. As a practical matter, OBRA 89 requires that the needs of the Medicare program and peer review organizations be considered by AHCPR in selecting topics for guidelines development, encouraging the dissemination and use of guidelines, and evaluating their impact. In addition, the agency must arrange for the development of medical review criteria and other practice evaluation tools. These factors appear sufficient to ensure that the needs of payers, consumer groups, and similar parties will be addressed during the guidelines development stage.

EVALUATION INSTRUMENTS

As defined above, practice guidelines are meant to assist patients and practitioners in making health care decisions. Medical review criteria, standards of quality, and performance measures, which the committee groups together as practice evaluation instruments, are designed to assist health care organizations, payers, and others (including practitioners and payers themselves) in evaluating those decisions and health outcomes. Sometimes such evaluations will focus on individual instances of care (for example, to determine whether a hysterectomy is appropriate for a patient with specific clinical characteristics); at other times they may focus on patterns of care (for example, to compare rates of hysterectomies for groups of patients with similar clinical characteristics).

Because the committee was not asked to provide principles for translating guidelines into evaluation instruments, it did not give in-depth consideration to the issues the Forum may face in moving from a given set of practice guidelines to the corresponding evaluation instruments. The committee did not, for example, discuss whether different principles and translation strategies might be needed for guidelines that focus heavily on nursing care compared to those that mainly emphasize care provided by physicians. The recent IOM report on quality assurance in the Medicare program (1990) discusses some of the attributes that good review criteria should have.

Given the expectations that guidelines will be used to improve the quality and effectiveness of health care, the task of clearly translating guidelines into evaluation tools is a critical one that needs to be considered during the process of guidelines development rather than at its end. At this early stage in the Forum's work, however, it may not be feasible for each set of guidelines to be accompanied by all three types of evaluation instruments.[5] As the Forum and its expert panels tackle specific decisions about evaluation instruments, they may well suggest some adjustments in the definitions offered below. This seems a possibility in particular for the definition of standards of quality and the provisional definition of performance measures, both of which gave the committee substantial difficulty in their formulation.

MEDICAL REVIEW CRITERIA

COMMON USAGE: THE DICTIONARY

According to the *Random House Dictionary*, a criterion is "a standard of judgment or criticism; a rule or principle for evaluating or testing something." The *OED* offers three definitions: an organ, faculty, or instrument of judging; a test, principle, rule, canon, or standard, by which anything is judged or estimated; and a distinguishing mark or characteristic, attaching to a thing, by which it can be judged or estimated.

---

[5] For the initial set of conditions for which guidelines are due by January 1, 1991, OBRA 89 is somewhat inconsistent about what is required of the Forum. Section 912(d) of the law (part of the amendments to the Public Health Service Act) calls for the development of guidelines, standards, performance measures, and review criteria, whereas section 1142(a)(3)(A) requires only guidelines.

PROFESSIONAL AND TECHNICAL USAGE

AMA (J. Kelly, director of the Office of Quality Assurance, letter dated April 26, 1990): Review criteria are "bases for evaluating quality and appropriateness of medical care."

IOM (1974:28): " 'Criteria' are identifiable elements of care used to judge the appropriateness of that care. . . ."

Professional Standards Review Organization (PSRO) Manual (cited in Donabedian, 1981): Medical care criteria are predetermined elements against which aspects of the quality of medical services may be compared.

Avedis Donabedian (1981:411): Although he apparently wishes to avoid use of the term *criterion*, Donabedian notes that it could usefully be employed to mean "an element or attribute that is to be used in evaluation, and that often comes accompanied by an explicit or implicit norm. . .or, even, by a standard." Elsewhere (p. 410), he says criteria are "discrete, clearly definable, and precisely measurable phenomena that belong within the categories of process or of outcome, and that, in some specifiable way, are relevant to the definition of quality."

Kathleen Lohr and Robert Brook (1981:761–762): "Quality-of-care criteria are commonly characterized in several ways. One is whether they are explicit (i.e., stated in detail in advance) or implicit (i.e., based on judgments of experts without direct reference to a priori standards). . . . Criteria may be thought of as minimal, average, or ideal. . . . [M]inimal criteria place a base under which the care-giver should not fall, lest the individual be judged as practicing severely substandard care. Those who fall below this level might well be classified as outliers. Average criteria represent a community standard; they are often thought of as a range within which care is considered acceptable. The lower bound [of average criteria] is likely to be the minimal point. . . . The upper bound is likely to be a fairly high, 'ideal' point toward which the profession may simply aspire."

Heather Palmer and Miriam Adams (forthcoming): Criteria are "predetermined elements of care against which aspects of the quality of a medical service may be compared." Prescriptive criteria are "criteria written by asking providers to decide what *ought* to be done in a given circumstance. Physicians writing such criteria have been found sometimes to specify care at an unrealistically high level. Also called normative criteria." (emphasis in the original)

Hannu Vuori (1989:156): "Criteria of good care are structural elements of care or procedures to be performed and information to be gathered when treating a patient with a given problem. . .or outcomes of care." Moreover, Vuori states that "criteria. . .identify the most important elements of good care. . . ."

THE COMMITTEE'S DEFINITION: MEDICAL REVIEW CRITERIA

Medical review criteria are systematically developed statements that can be used to assess the appropriateness of specific health care decisions, services, and outcomes.

For medical review criteria, the committee definition stresses the *evaluation* of health care processes and outcomes rather than assistance to practitioners and patients in making decisions. The definition offered here is reasonably consistent with legislative language and most professional and common usage. It is also reasonably succinct and not tautological. As noted earlier in this chapter, the committee's definition of appropriate care does not require that judgments be made about the cost-effectiveness of particular clinical practices.[6] Neither does the definition preclude it.

Medical review criteria have many different uses and users. They may be used (1) prospectively, for example, to review a proposed hospital admission or surgical procedure; (2) concurrently, for instance, to assess the need for continued hospitalization; or (3) retrospectively, for example, to make decisions about insurance claims. Criteria-based reviews may focus on patterns of practice or on individual cases of care. For example, reviewers concerned primarily with assessing the quality of care may concentrate on retrospective analyses of patterns of care; they may also rely heavily on case-finding screens applied retrospectively to identify individual potential problems for further evaluation using more detailed criteria (IOM, 1990). Users more concerned with cost management have increasingly emphasized review criteria that can be applied prospectively on a case-by-case basis to certain relatively expensive procedures (IOM, 1989).

Traditional criteria for judging the process of care most often specify only the things that should be done and ignore things that should not be done. In contrast, criteria used for insurance claims review tend to screen for the inappropriate service rather than list everything that is appropriate. (Claims review may also include a variety of nonclinical matters, such as whether the general category of service, setting, and provider was covered under a patient's benefit plan and whether the service was correctly coded.)

As noted earlier, some practice guidelines may translate into or be used as medical review criteria in a straightforward fashion (just as some foreign words and phrases—for example, caveat emptor—are easily used by English speakers). For practical or technical reasons, other guidelines may be more difficult or less suitable for use in this way. Of the initial conditions being

---

[6] A recent IOM report (1989) noted that most private payers and review organizations claim that their retrospective reviews of care for specific patients focus on clinical factors, not costs, and that their emphasis is on detecting clearly inappropriate care.

considered by the Forum for guidelines development (see the list presented in Chapter 1), the agency may find, for example, that medical review criteria are easier to develop from the cataracts guidelines than from the guidelines for treatment of depression in the community setting. Similarly, the guidelines for managing incontinence may give rise to criteria for reviewing quality but none for making payment decisions.

STANDARDS OF QUALITY

The term *standards* is particularly difficult to clarify. In common parlance it is often used synonymously with criteria; in the quality assurance lexicon, however, it has rather different connotations. Even in everyday use, *standard* has many different senses.

COMMON USAGE: THE DICTIONARY

The *Random House Dictionary* offers more than 25 meanings including the following: "1. something considered by an authority or by general consent as a basis of comparison; an approved model. . . 3. a rule or principle that is used as a basis for judgment. . . 4. an average or normal requirement, quality, quantity, level, grade, etc. . . . 24. of recognized excellence or established authority; and 25. usual, common, customary." This dictionary suggests that a standard differs from a criterion in that the former implies a model against which the quality or excellence of other things may be determined ("she could serve as the standard of good breeding") whereas the latter does not ("wealth is not a criterion of a person's worth").

The *OED* sets forth the following different meanings and definition for *standard* (some of which are centuries old): "1. the exemplar of a measure or weight; 2. a normal uniform size or amount; a prescribed minimum size or amount; 3. an authoritative or recognized exemplar of correctness, perfection, or some definite degree of any quality (which can be construed as a rule, principle, or means of judgment or estimation, or a criterion or measure); and 4. a definite level of excellence, attainment, wealth, or the like, or a definite degree of any quality, viewed as a prescribed object of endeavour or as the measure of what is adequate for some purpose."

The most troublesome aspect of common usage is the use of *standard* in quite different ways to describe either a minimum acceptable state or a state of high achievement and excellence. The same difficulty also shows up in the health services literature.

PROFESSIONAL AND TECHNICAL USAGE

AMA (J. Kelly, director of the Office of Quality Assurance, letter dated April 26, 1990): A standard is an "accepted principle for patient management."

IOM (1974:28): "A 'standard' is the degree of adherence to the defined criteria."

Joint Commission on Accreditation of Healthcare Organizations (1989a): "expectations or rules relating to the structures or processes necessary for delivery of patient care."

PSRO Manual (cited in Donabedian, 1981): "Standards are professionally developed expressions of the range of acceptable variation from a norm or criterion."

Mark Chassin (1988:438–439): Chassin refers to "standards of care or practice guidelines" and goes on to say that "[t]hey can also define several levels of quality of care, from the best attainable to a minimal level below which care is unacceptably poor. They can also be applied to groups of patients as well as to individuals."

David Eddy (forthcoming): In distinguishing standards, guidelines, and options for "practice policies," Eddy makes the following point: "A practice policy is considered a standard if the health and economic consequences of an intervention are sufficiently well known to permit meaningful decisions and there is virtual unanimity among patients about the desirability (or undesirability) of the intervention, and about the proper use (or nonuse) of the intervention." (That is, a standard is the most stringent form of a practice policy.)

Heather Palmer and Miriam Adams (forthcoming): Standards are "professionally developed expressions of the range of acceptable variation from norms or criteria." Palmer goes on to say "commonly, all-or-nothing standards (for example, 100 percent or 0 percent compliance required) are preferred. This is coupled with peer review of all cases that vary from the criteria."

Virgil Slee (1974): "The *desired* achievable (rather than the *observed*) performance or value with regard to a given parameter." (emphasis in original) *Parameter* is then defined as "an objective, definable, and measurable characteristic of the patient himself or of the process or outcome of his care. Each parameter has a scale of possible values. . . ."

Hannu Vuori (1989:156): "A standard is the value of a criterion that indicates the border between acceptable and poor quality. Standards can be normative or empirical.[7] A normative standard equates the acceptable performance with either the best imaginable performance or the best attainable performance under ideal circumstances. Empirical standards are

---

[7] Connotations derived from "norm" and "normative" cause endless problems. Some experts,

often based on experiences gained in 'typical' situations." In addition, Vuori states that "standards. . .indicate which level [of a criterion] should be reached. . . ."

THE COMMITTEE'S DEFINITION: STANDARDS OF QUALITY

Standards of quality are authoritative statements of (1) minimum levels of acceptable performance or results, (2) excellent levels of performance or results, *or* (3) the range of acceptable performance or results.

Given the contradictory uses of the term, the committee decided it was pointless to try to overrule them. Instead, it takes the position that clarity about the nature of a standard is the key issue: does the standard *clearly* state that it sets a minimum level of performance or a level of excellence or a range? Preferably, specific labels such as "minimal standards" or "standards of excellence" should be employed.

Defining standards of quality will be a major enterprise. Another IOM report, *Medicare: A Strategy for Quality Assurance* (1990), provides an extensive overview of quality assurance activities, methods, and problems and recommends a 10-year strategy for improving the country's quality assessment and assurance efforts and results. In that report, quality of care is defined as "the degree to which health services for individuals and populations increase the likelihood of desired health outcomes and are consistent with current professional knowledge" (p. 4). One point made about this definition is that it "encompasses a wide range of elements of care." This suggests that standards of quality should be viewed primarily as means for assessing *patterns* of care, including patterns that may extend across a range of clinical conditions, settings, and practitioners.

Advice about whether the Forum should emphasize minimum standards or standards of excellence or ranges is beyond the scope of this report. Among other things, such advice would entail an analysis of alternative views about how to assure quality of care. For example, the concept of minimum standards seems more consistent with the structure-process-outcome model of quality assurance than the continuous quality improvement model. The 1990 IOM report cited above discusses these models at some length, but that discussion provides no simple path for this committee to follow in specifically advising the Forum. Such advice

---

including Vuori and Palmer, see norms as ideal or preferred states. Others treat norm and "average" as essentially equivalent, and they equate the normative and the empirical because empirical data are needed to determine "norms." A 1974 IOM report, for instance, defined "norm" as "merely a statistical average" (p. 28).

might also be premature, given that the Department of Health and Human Services and Congress are considering a variety of policy and strategy issues related to broad questions of quality assurance and assessment. Decisions on these issues presumably should influence the Forum's work.

PERFORMANCE MEASURES

This concept is the most unfamiliar of the four terms in OBRA 89. It is seldom used in the professional literature and has a variety of dictionary definitions.

COMMON USAGE: THE DICTIONARY

Random House offers for performance "the manner in which or the efficiency with which something reacts or fulfills its intended purpose." The *OED* provides two relevant definitions for performance: "1. the carrying out of a demand, duty, purpose, promise, etc.; 2. the accomplishment, execution, . . .of anything ordered or undertaken."

The *OED* gives many different definitions for measure. As a verb, these include "1. to form an estimate of (now especially to weigh or gauge the character or ability of something [e.g., a person]), with a view to what to expect [from that person]; 2. to ascertain or determine the spatial magnitude or quantity of [something] by application or comparison to some known or fixed unit; 3. to estimate the amount, duration, value, etc., of an immaterial thing [perhaps, performance] by comparison with some standard; 4. to judge or estimate the greatness or value of (a person, a quality) by a certain standard or rule; and to appraise by comparison with something else." As a noun, the definitions of measure include "1. an instrument for measuring [e.g., a vessel, graduated rod, line, tape, etc. . . .]; and 2. a method of measuring, especially a system of standard denomination of units of length [etc.]."

PROFESSIONAL AND TECHNICAL USAGE

The term *performance measure* has been used by the Joint Commission on Accreditation of Healthcare Organizations, but the commission intends, in the future, to substitute the term *indicator* (R. Marder, project manager, Indicator Development, personal communication, April 24, 1990). Committee staff found virtually no discussion of performance measures in the literature they reviewed.

Joint Commission (1989b:4–5): "Performance measures provide data and information that serve as the basis for determining whether expectations are met." A clinical indicator is a "generic term. . .intended to emphasize

the primary importance of (outcome) measures as monitors of performance.
... [They] describe relatively precise measures of important aspects of care.
... [They] are not clinical standards or practice guidelines."

David Eddy (forthcoming): In discussing the distinction between practice policies (see the earlier section) and performance policies, he notes that performance policies address the issue of ensuring that "whatever interventions are used, are used correctly. . . . They are intended to guide or review the performance of interventions, without concern for whether the interventions should have been performed in the first place."

THE COMMITTEE'S PROVISIONAL DEFINITION: PERFORMANCE MEASURES

Performance measures are methods or instruments to estimate or monitor the extent to which the actions of a health care practitioner or provider conform to practice guidelines, medical review criteria, or standards of quality.

Given the multiple common meanings of the term and the paucity of professional and technical usage, the committee decided to offer only a provisional definition of performance measures. As practice guidelines and related evaluation instruments are more widely developed and used, a different or more specific meaning for this term may emerge.

The committee could have considered performance measures to be a combination of standards and criteria—measures of whether a given "performance" as judged by some set of criteria meets (or exceeds or falls short of) a standard. Considered in this way, the term verges on being synonymous with the other terms defined in this chapter. Therefore, the committee chose provisionally to view performance measures as instruments (for example, questionnaires, abstracting forms, measurement scales, or computer programs) for recording or measuring data on performance. In this sense, a distinction is made between measuring and judging. Thus, a performance measure is more like a bathroom scale than it is like a table of recommended weights by gender and body build.

In sum, it is probably valuable to maintain a distinction between the instrument or means of measuring something and the judging of the results. Furthermore, performance measures should be sensitive to what is *not* done as well as what is done.

CONCLUSIONS AND SUMMARY

In this chapter, the committee has proposed definitions of the four key terms used in the legislation establishing the Office of the Forum for Quality and Effectiveness in Health Care. The committee sought definitions that were, insofar as possible, parsimonious, consistent with common and professional usage, practically and symbolically acceptable to important interests, not easily misused, and not tautological. The list below recapitulates the committee's definitions of practice guidelines, medical review criteria, standards of quality, and performance measures.

• **PRACTICE GUIDELINES** are systematically developed statements to assist practitioner and patient decisions about appropriate health care for specific clinical circumstances.

• **MEDICAL REVIEW CRITERIA** are systematically developed statements that can be used to assess the appropriateness of specific health care decisions, services, and outcomes.

• **STANDARDS OF QUALITY** are authoritative statements of (1) minimum levels of acceptable performance or results, (2) excellent levels of performance or results, *or* (3) the range of acceptable performance or results.

• **PERFORMANCE MEASURES** (provisional) are methods or instruments to estimate or monitor the extent to which the actions of a health care practitioner or provider conform to practice guidelines, medical review criteria, or standards of quality.

For other organizations and other purposes, different terms and definitions may serve better as long as they are clearly stated. This committee neither expects nor wishes to dictate terminology. Its objective is modest: to provide clear definitions of key terms that the Forum can use in carrying out its legal responsibilities with a minimum of confusion or provocation.

Definitions, however, are only the starting point. The Forum also needs to distinguish good guidelines from bad and to communicate its expectations to contractors, expert panels, and others. The next chapter is a first step in that process.

REFERENCES

Chassin, M.R. Standards of Care in Medicine. *Inquiry* 25(Winter):437–450, 1988.
Compact Edition of the Oxford English Dictionary. Oxford, England: Oxford University Press, 1971.
Donabedian, A. Criteria, Norms and Standards of Quality: What Do They Mean? *American Journal of Public Health* 71:409–412, 1981.
Eddy, D. *A Manual for Assessing Health Practices and Designing Practice Policies* (draft dated May 31, 1989). American College of Physicians, forthcoming. See also the articles cited in Chapter 1 of this report.
Havighurst, C. Practice Guidelines for Medical Care: The Policy Rationale. *St. Louis University Law Journal,* forthcoming.
Institute of Medicine. *Advancing the Quality of Health Care.* Washington, D.C.: National Academy Press, 1974.

Institute of Medicine. *Controlling Costs and Changing Patient Care? The Role of Utilization Management*, B. Gray and M. Field, eds. Washington, D.C.: National Academy Press, 1989.

Institute of Medicine. *Medicare: A Strategy for Quality Assurance*, vols. 1 and 2, K. Lohr, ed., Washington, D.C.: National Academy Press, 1990.

Joint Commission on Accreditation of Healthcare Organizations. A National Invitational Forum on Clinical Indicator Development, Chicago, March 1989a.

Joint Commission on Accreditation of Healthcare Organizations. Statement before the House Subcommittee on Health, Committee on Ways and Means, concerning the Medical Care Quality Research Act of 1989. Washington, D.C., May 24, 1989b.

Leape, L. Practice Guidelines and Standards: An Overview. *Quality Review Bulletin* 16:42–49, 1990.

Lohr, K.N., and Brook, R.H. Quality Assurance and Clinical Pharmacy: Lessons from Medicine. *Drug Intelligence and Clinical Pharmacy* 15:758–765, 1981.

Meyer, H. Medicine Debates Parameters (Or Are They Guidelines?). *American Medical News*, December 15, 1989, p. 36.

Palmer, R.H., and Adams, M. Considerations in Defining Quality of Health Care. In *Perspectives on Quality Assurance*. Ann Arbor, Mich.: Health Administration Press, forthcoming.

Park, R.E., Fink, A., Brook, R.H., et al. *Physician Ratings of Appropriate Indications for Six Medical and Surgical Procedures*. R-3280-CWF/HF/PMT/RWJ. Santa Monica, Calif.: The RAND Corporation, 1986.

Physician Payment Review Commission. Improving the Quality of Care: Clinical Research and Practice Guidelines. Appendix 1, Background Paper for Conference, October 1988; draft dated September 28, 1988a.

Physician Payment Review Commission. Increasing Appropriate Use of Services: Practice Guidelines and Feedback of Practice Patterns. Chapter 13 in *Annual Report to Congress*. Washington, D.C., 1988b.

Random House Dictionary of the English Language, 2nd ed., unabridged. New York: Random House, 1987.

Slee, V. PSRO and the Hospital's Quality Control. *Annals of Internal Medicine* 81:97–106, 1974; cited in Donabedian (1981).

U.S. Preventive Services Task Force. *Guide to Clinical Preventive Services: An Assessment of the Effectiveness of 169 Interventions*. Baltimore, Md.: Williams & Wilkins, 1989.

Vuori, H. Research Needs in Quality Assurance. *Quality Assurance in Health Care* 1:147–159, 1989.

3

Attributes of Good Practice Guidelines

Remember the drunk who searched for his keys under the lamp post because that's where the light was? Science is a highly systematic process of creating lamps and then looking under them.

David Warsh, *Washington Post*

Developing practice guidelines that enlighten practitioners and patients is an exceptionally challenging task. It requires diverse skills ranging from the analysis of scientific evidence to the management of group decisionmaking to the presentation of complex information in useful forms. Although the need for these skills has not always been recognized in the past, the recent focus on guidelines is bringing not only a greater awareness of what is required for their development but also a higher level of expertise to the field. The Office of the Forum for Quality and Effectiveness in Health Care should make every effort to reinforce this trend as it works with contractors, expert panels, and others to develop and disseminate practice guidelines.

This chapter describes eight attributes that the committee believes are essential if a set of guidelines are to serve their intended purposes of assisting practitioners and patients, providing a better foundation for the evaluation of services and practitioners, and improving health outcomes. These attributes are ideal characteristics to which real guidelines are unlikely to conform fully either now or in the future. However, in the committee's judgment, guidelines can approach these ideals to a greater extent than has generally been achieved to date.

The next four sections review the context, working assumptions, principles, and sources that guided the committee in developing its list of attributes, followed by a discussion of the attributes themselves. This chapter, however, is not intended either as an exhaustive description of how guidelines should be developed or as an endorsement of one specific method.[1] The discussion in this chapter focuses on attributes of guidelines rather than attributes of medical review criteria, standards of quality, and performance measures. The recent IOM report on quality assurance in the Medicare program (1990d) discusses some attributes that good medical review criteria should have, for example, specificity and sensitivity.

One further introductory point: the committee has urged AHCPR and its Forum to focus their efforts on guidelines for clinical conditions rather than specific treatments or procedures. This focus will undoubtedly make their task more difficult: a consideration of conditions generally involves a broader look at alternatives, evidence, practice settings, and outcomes. The result, however, should be guidelines that are both more broadly *and* more specifically useful to clinicians and patients. The discussion of attributes in this chapter reflects this emphasis on conditions rather than procedures.

BACKGROUND AND TERMINOLOGY

OBRA 89 specifies that "the Director [of the Forum] shall establish standards and criteria to be utilized by the recipients of contracts" for "developing and periodically reviewing and updating" guidelines, standards, performance measures, and review criteria. Confusion is likely if "criteria and standards" are used to label both the bases for prospectively assessing practice guidelines and the bases for assessing clinician practice. Consequently, to reduce possible terminological confusion, this report refers to "attributes of guidelines" rather than to "standards and criteria" for "guidelines, standards, performance measures, and review criteria." Synonyms include properties and characteristics.[2]

The Forum must be able to employ the list of attributes set forth in this chapter in at least two ways. First, it will need to communicate its expectations *in advance* to the contractors or expert panels that may develop guidelines for the agency. Second, the Forum and potential users of the guidelines must be able to assess the soundness of a given set of guidelines *after* they are developed. The IOM expects in a second project

---

[1] The list of works by Eddy, Gottlieb and associates, and Park and colleagues at the end of this chapter contains more detailed discussions of processes for developing guidelines.

[2] This language generally follows the precedent set by the IOM report *Medicare: A Strategy for Quality Assurance* (1990d). It is also consistent with the booklet "Attributes to Guide the Development of Practice Parameters" (AMA, 1990a).

to prepare a practical assessment instrument that the Forum can use to systematically review guidelines developed by its panels or by other groups (Appendix C).

During the committee's deliberations, a question was raised about whether the Forum has formal authority under OBRA 89 either to reject or approve the guidelines developed by its contractors or expert panels. This report does not speak to that legal point. Nevertheless, regardless of the Forum's statutory authority in this regard, it is reasonable that the agency should examine the soundness of guidelines developed under its auspices. This examination may (1) improve the way the agency works with contractors or panels in the future, (2) contribute to more informed consideration of dissemination options and evaluation strategies, (3) allow more sophisticated consultations with HCFA and other government agencies about their use of the guidelines, and (4) provide feedback about the feasibility of the assessments proposed here.

In this report, *assessment* means the prospective or initial judgment of the soundness and feasibility of a set of guidelines. In contrast, the empirical *evaluation* of the cost, quality, and other effects of guidelines occurs after they are published and implemented.

Further, a *set* of guidelines includes a series of statements or recommendations about appropriate practice and the accompanying descriptions of evidence, methodology, and rationale. A guideline in the singular refers to a discrete statement or recommendation (for example, annual breast physical examination for women aged 40 to 49 with no family or personal history of breast cancer). Each of the appropriateness reports published by the RAND Corporation clearly exemplifies a set of guidelines (Park et al., 1986). Likewise, using this terminology, the report of the U.S. Preventive Services Task Force (1989) contains 60 sets of guidelines and not 60 guidelines.

WORKING ASSUMPTIONS

The committee's first working assumption has been that a set of guidelines will be assessed as a whole; that is, its elements will not be assessed individually in isolation. Under this assumption the Forum could judge a set of guidelines acceptable even if individual statements lacked—for legitimate reasons—some essential attributes. Realistically, early guidelines and (especially) existing guidelines are not likely to score well on all eight attributes collectively. However, the committee expects that, as the development process matures, guidelines will continue to comprise more and more of the attributes.

Second, the committee assumes that the Forum will (in line with OBRA 89 provisions) convene expert panels to assess either existing guidelines or guidelines for which the Forum has contracted. These panels will need to make both objective and subjective assessments guided by instructions from the Forum. This report is a step toward the preparation of an assessment instrument that the expert panels can use in their reviews and deliberations (Appendix C). The AMA has recently taken a similar step by developing a preliminary worksheet to evaluate what it terms practice parameters (AMA, 1990b).

Third, the committee sees the initial assessment of guidelines as part of an evolutionary process of guidelines development, assessment, use, evaluation, and revision. This evolutionary process will involve the government, professional organizations, health service researchers, consumers, and others. As a result, the committee fully expects the set of attributes presented here to be tested, reassessed, and revised, if necessary.

PRINCIPLES

The identification of attributes of practice guidelines rests on four principles. These principles call for:

- *clarity* in the definition of each attribute;
- *compatibility* of each attribute and its definition with professional usage;
- *clear rationales or justifications* for the selection of each attribute; and
- *sensitivity to practical issues* in using the attributes to assess actual sets of practice guidelines ("assessibility").

That the definition of an attribute be clear and succinct is obviously desirable, although often difficult when one is working with very abstract or technical concepts. It is also desirable that the term used to label an attribute be recognizable and consistent with customary professional usage. The label should be a single word or short phrase that is carefully chosen to convey the core concept. (Thus, attributes will not be described by number, for example, Attribute No. 1.)

The rationale or justification for each attribute should be clearly described, and it should also be consistent with the professional and technical literature and the legislative mandate. The rationale should describe explicitly any trade-offs between the theoretically ideal attribute and the practical, usable one.

Practicality requires that attributes be definable in operational as well as conceptual terms; that is, it should be possible to devise an instrument that instructs assessors of a set of guidelines on how they can determine whether the guidelines conform to the attributes. Not only is this necessary if the Forum is to judge the soundness of the guidelines that emerge from its expert panels; it is fundamental that the Forum instruct developers of guidelines on the desired properties of guidelines and on the documentation needed as a basis for assessment. As mentioned earlier, the development of a formal instrument for assessing guidelines is an important next step for this committee.

More generally, the number of attributes must be sensible and practical. An appropriate balance must be reached between enough attributes to allow adequate assessment of the guidelines but not so many that the assessment exercise becomes infeasible, confusing, or excessive, given limited resources. It is likely that an instrument for assessing guidelines will need to *weight* the eight attributes in some manner, specifying which of them are more significant in determining whether a given set of guidelines are sound. Given its time and resource constraints, this committee did not systematically rank the different attributes by relative importance, although the discussion below does distinguish some of the more important ones.

A final point: this report differentiates between the *priorities* for selecting particular targets for guidelines and the desirable *attributes* of guidelines. The attributes listed in this chapter do not incorporate the OBRA 89 provisions requiring that priorities for the development of guidelines reflect the needs and priorities of the Medicare program and include clinical treatments or conditions accounting for a significant portion of Medicare expenditures.

The legislation also calls on the Secretary of Health and Human Services to consider the extent to which guidelines can be expected "(i) to improve methods of prevention, diagnosis, treatment, and clinical management for the benefit of a significant number of individuals; (ii) to reduce clinically significant variations among physicians in the particular services and procedures utilized in making diagnoses and providing treatment; and (iii) to reduce clinically significant variations in the outcomes of health care services and procedures." In arriving at its eight recommended properties of guidelines, the committee did not incorporate these factors. Priority setting is a crucial but separate task and one that IOM has undertaken as part of other studies (IOM, 1990a,b,c,e).

PAST WORK ON DEFINING ATTRIBUTES

This committee considered three primary sources in identifying attributes for practice guidelines: (1) the legislation, (2) the IOM report on quality assurance for Medicare, and (3) work by the AMA. Other important materials, which in some cases were used in the primary sources, include the work of Brook, Chassin, Eddy, Greenfield, and their collaborators, as cited elsewhere in this report.

In addition to describing priorities to guide the Forum in selecting topics for guidelines, OBRA 89 sets forth some characteristics that guidelines should have. The committee distinguished these four points from the legislation.

1. Guidelines should be based on the best available research and professional judgment regarding the effectiveness and appropriateness of health care services and procedures.

2. The Forum director is expected to ensure that appropriate, interested individuals and organizations will be consulted during the development of guidelines.

3. The director has the power to pilot-test the guidelines.

4. Guidelines should be presented in forms appropriate for use in clinical practice, in educational programs, and in reviewing quality and appropriateness of medical care.

A second major source for the committee's work, the IOM report on a quality assurance strategy for Medicare (1990d), included a chapter on attributes of quality of care and appropriateness criteria. These attributes derived from a June 1989 meeting of experts on the construction and use of practice guidelines. Some of the distinctions proposed by the quality panel are not used here. For example, this committee's report emphasizes key attributes of good guidelines but contains relatively little discussion of desirable but less critical attributes. In addition, this report drops the panel's distinction between substantive and implementation guidelines because the committee found it awkward to label every attribute as either one or the other. The point that lay behind the original distinction should, nonetheless, be stressed: the designers of guidelines need to keep implementation in mind—whether and how the guidelines can be used.

A third source considered by the committee was the AMA's booklet, "Attributes to Guide the Development of Practice Parameters" (1990a), which sets forth five attributes. They are (minus their accompanying discussion and more detailed descriptions) as follows: (1) practice parameters should be developed by or in conjunction with physician organizations; (2) reliable methodologies that integrate relevant research findings and appropriate clinical expertise should be used to develop practice parameters; (3) practice parameters should be as comprehensive and specific as possible; (4) practice parameters should be based on current information; and (5) practice parameters should be widely distributed.

ATTRIBUTES FOR ASSESSING PRACTICE GUIDELINES: OVERVIEW

The art of developing practice guidelines is in an early stage, and the strengths and weaknesses of specific approaches are still being debated. As a consequence, the committee recognizes that what is expected of guidelines, in terms of their development and implementation, will need to evolve beyond these initial specifications.

Table 3-1 lists the eight attributes for assessing guidelines that the committee identified. One theme emphasized here, which ties these guideline attributes together, is *credibility*—credibility with practitioners, with patients, with payers, with policymakers. This theme encompasses the scientific grounding of the guidelines, the qualifications of those involved in the development process, and the relevance of the guidelines to the actual world in which practitioners and patients make decisions.

A second and related theme is the importance of *accountability*, a key element of which is disclosure. That is, the committee expects that procedures, participants, evidence, assumptions, rationales, and analytic methods will be meticulously documented—preferably in an accompanying background paper. This documentation will help those not participating in any given process of guidelines formulation to assess independently the soundness of the developers' work.

Explanations should be provided for any conflict or inconsistency between the guidelines in question and those developed by others. The issue of disagreement or inconsistency among practice guidelines is an important one for patients, practitioners, managers, payers, and policymakers. As discussed in Chapter 5 of this report, merely identifying inconsistencies in guidelines says nothing about the legitimacy of such differences. Careful documentation of the evidence and rationales can help potential users of guidelines judge whether inconsistencies arise from differences in the interpretation of scientific evidence, from differences in the care taken in developing the guidelines, or from other factors.

VALIDITY

In the committee's view, the validity of practice guidelines ranks as the most critical attribute, even though it may be the hardest to define and measure. Conceptually, a valid practice guideline is one that, if followed, will lead to the health and cost outcomes projected for it, other things being equal. In the research literature, validity is commonly defined by three questions. Do the instruments for measuring some concept (for example, quality of care) really measure that concept? Does the relationship or effect that the researchers assert exists (for example, following a set of guidelines improves quality of care) really exist? Can that relationship be generalized (for example, from clinical trials to everyday medical practice)?

Until a guideline is actually applied and the results evaluated, validity must be assessed primarily by reference to the substance and quality of the evidence cited, the means used to evaluate the evidence, and the

TABLE 3-1 Eight Attributes of Good Practice Guidelines

Attribute	Discussion
Validity	Practice guidelines are valid if, when followed, they lead to the health and cost outcomes projected for them, other things being equal. A prospective assessment of validity will consider the projected health outcomes and costs of alternative courses of action, the relationship between the evidence and recommendations, the substance and quality of the scientific and clinical evidence cited, and the means used to evaluate the evidence.
Reliability/ reproducibility	Practice guidelines are reliable and reproducible (1) if—given the same evidence and methods for guidelines development—another set of experts would produce essentially the same statements and (2) if—given the same clinical circumstances—the guidelines are interpreted and applied consistently by practitioners or other appropriate parties. A prospective assessment of reliability may consider the results of independent external reviews and pretests of the guidelines.
Clinical applicability	Practice guidelines should be as inclusive of appropriately defined patient populations as scientific and clinical evidence and expert judgment permit, and they should explicitly state the populations to which statements apply.
Clinical flexibility	Practice guidelines should identify the specifically known or generally expected exceptions to their recommendations.
Clarity	Practice guidelines should use unambiguous language, define terms precisely, and use logical, easy-to-follow modes of presentation.
Multidisciplinary process	Practice guidelines should be developed by a process that includes participation by representatives of key affected groups. Participation may include serving on panels that develop guidelines, providing evidence and viewpoints to the panels, and reviewing draft guidelines.
Scheduled review	Practice guidelines should include statements about when they should be reviewed to determine whether revisions are warranted, given new clinical evidence or changing professional consensus.
Documentation	The procedures followed in developing guidelines, the participants involved, the evidence used, the assumptions and rationales accepted, and the analytic methods employed should be meticulously documented and described.

relationship between the evidence and recommendations.[3] In the context of the Forum's practical needs, the committee recommends that an assessment of validity look for 11 elements in a set of guidelines. These elements are listed below:

- Projected health outcomes
- Projected costs
- Relationship between the evidence and the guidelines
- Preference for empirical evidence over expert judgment
- Thorough literature review
- Methods used to evaluate the scientific literature
- Strength of the evidence
- Use of expert judgment
- Strength of expert consensus
- Independent review
- Pretesting.

PROJECTED HEALTH OUTCOMES

A key reason for developing and using practice guidelines is the expectation that they will improve health outcomes. Ideally, a set of guidelines should give practitioners, patients, and policymakers an explicit description of the projected health benefits (for example, a reduction in postoperative infection rates from 4 to 2 percent) and the projected harms or risks (for example, an increase in the risk of incontinence from 10 to 20 percent). If reasonable and technically feasible, the *net* effects of a course of action—the balance of benefits against risks or harms—also need to be estimated. In addition, projected outcomes should be compared with those for alternative courses of care for the clinical condition in question.

The ideal set of projections just described will often be technically or practically beyond the reach of guidelines developers. In most situations, the assistance of outside consultants or specialized technical advisory panels will be at least helpful or at most essential; yet even with such help, projecting health outcomes is intrinsically a complex and subjective process. The nature of the process makes it particularly important that the methods

---

[3] The committee discussed four types of validity: face validity, content validity, criterion validity, and construct validity. These concepts may have the following connotations when applied to practice guidelines. First, the content of guidelines and their development processes need to be plausible, at first pass, to practitioners—to have *face validity*. Second, *content validity* has to be assessed by reviewing the scientific evidence on which a set of guidelines are based—how much evidence there is, how clear it is, how directly it relates to the guidelines, how sound its methodology is. Third, for a prospective assessment of *criterion validity*, one judges whether the guidelines would be likely to produce predicted results when applied in the real world of health care delivery. *Construct validity* involves the fit of the guideline to broader scientific theories.

INFORMATION ABOUT CLINICAL BENEFITS AND ABOUT RISKS OR HARMS

1. What are the potential benefits and risks (type and importance) for individual patients associated with an intervention or procedure?
2. What is the probability that a benefit or harm will occur?
3. Do benefits exceed harms? By how much?
4. What characteristics of delivery settings or patients affect the probability of a benefit or harm?
5. How are benefits and harms distributed across time and populations?
6. How do these benefits and harms compare for alternative practices?

INFORMATION ABOUT COSTS AND SAVINGS

1. What is the production cost/price of a particular test, intervention, etc.? What are other important costs, such as for program administration?
2. What is the total cost, given the projected number of services provided?
3. What is the cost per unit of some benefit, including not only the immediate cost of providing service but the cost of follow-up services (for example, the cost of screening for cancer and the cost of treating cancers that are detected)?
4. What costs may be averted or saved (individual, total)?
5. How do costs and savings compare for alternative courses of action?

FIGURE 3-1 A possible checklist for describing benefits, risks, and costs. SOURCE: This figure is adapted in part from the National Research Council report, *Improving Risk Communication* (1989).

for projecting outcomes, the limitations in these methods, and the evidence for such projections be described.

When empirical evidence is limited, potential effects may only be listed, not quantitatively compared or weighed. In addition, in cases in which patient preferences about different risks and benefits may differ, practice guidelines will need to be sensitive to such variation, and a comprehensive statement of net effects may have to be omitted (Mulley, 1990). In any event, a systematic effort should be made to provide practitioners, patients, and others with information that will help them make their own judgments of the balance of benefits and risks.

Figure 3-1 provides a simple checklist of outcomes that might be estimated. The particular outcomes to be considered will vary with the clinical conditions and practices under consideration.

To support the eventual evaluation of the actual impact of guidelines, guidelines developers should indicate what information related to outcomes will be needed, where it can be obtained, and whether better means for collecting and analyzing data need to be established to permit evaluation.

On this last point, limitations in the sources of data and the variables used to project outcomes are likely to provide inspiration for recommending improvements.

PROJECTED COSTS

Recent interest in practice guidelines is founded in part on the explicit or implicit expectation that they can help control escalating health care costs. The committee has already cautioned that some guidelines, if followed, may increase short- or long-term costs and that the net cost effects of current initiatives are not clear. These kinds of uncertainty underscore the desirability of including some form of cost projections in the background documentation for guidelines.

Cost estimation, like the projection of health outcomes, has its own special technical complexities and subjective aspects that will often require the services of outside consultants or specialized technical advisory panels. Even with such assistance, the committee recognizes that the results will be imperfect. In general, estimates of the costs associated with a set of guidelines should follow the same principles of documentation and discussion described for the estimation of health outcomes, including comparisons of alternative courses of care (see Figure 3-1). The remainder of this section describes desirable elements of cost projections, elements the committee sees as goals rather than minimum requirements.

Ideally, cost estimates should have two components, one involving projected health care costs and the other relating to administrative costs. The estimated health care costs of following the guidelines should reflect (1) the estimated total number of services that will be added, substituted, or deleted if a guideline is followed and (2) the substantiated charges (or production costs) for these services. For example, for screening services, the expected costs of providing the services and of treating the problems that are detected all need to be included. Depending on the available information and the assumptions used, estimates will often take the form of ranges rather than point estimates.

If health outcomes are projected in terms of additional life expectancy or similar measures, then the cost per unit of each identified outcome should be projected. Again, ranges may be more suitable than point estimates. If the guidelines indicate acceptable alternative courses of care, the total costs of the major alternatives and their cost per unit of each expected benefit should be described.

Cost estimates should also consider the additional expenses that may be associated with administering or using the guidelines. For example, computer hardware or software may be required to support easy access to various sets of guidelines. In the case of medical review criteria, additional staff may be required to handle inquiries.

This report does not take a position on whether costs should be explicitly factored into recommendations, although some committee members have strong views that such a step should be mandatory if guidelines are to control costs. The committee did agree that information on projected health outcomes and costs will help developers and users of guidelines better understand the implications of following or not following the guidelines. One part of this process will be some clarification of both the factual and the value judgments involved for practitioners, patients, health plans, and others in making such decisions. In some cases, a patient may decide that a service is not worth the personal out-of-pocket cost; in others, a provider may choose among clinically acceptable alternatives on the basis of financial considerations, such as the opportunity cost of acquiring new equipment. Similarly, a health benefits plan may opt not to cover a category of service that it is quite appropriate for a practitioner to provide and a patient to receive.[4]

RELATIONSHIP BETWEEN THE EVIDENCE AND THE GUIDELINES

Practice guidelines have not always been clearly and consistently related to the scientific and clinical evidence (Eddy and Billings, 1988), but they should be. The link between the base of evidence and a set of guidelines needs to be explicit, preferably with specific citations for specific portions of a set of guidelines. This implies the need for a reference list rather than just a bibliography of literature used in the guidelines development process. A bibliography may, however, indicate sources consulted but not cited.

PREFERENCE FOR EMPIRICAL EVIDENCE OVER EXPERT JUDGMENT

Empirical evidence should take precedence over expert judgment in the development of guidelines. When the empirical evidence has important limitations and experts reach conclusions that are not consistent with the evidence, then the conflict and limits of the evidence should be clearly described and the rationale for departing from the evidence, such as it is, should be explained. When expert judgment proceeds in the absence of

---

[4] For example, childhood immunizations and other preventive services have traditionally been excluded from indemnity health plans because insurers believe it is actuarially unwise to cover smaller, more predictable expenses that their subscribers can budget. Competitive pressures from health maintenance organizations may sometimes offset these beliefs, but this may reflect marketing more than clinical considerations.

direct empirical evidence about a particular clinical practice, a frequent circumstance, the general scientific reasoning or normative (ethical, professional) principles supporting the expert judgments should be described.

THOROUGH LITERATURE REVIEW

A thorough review of the scientific literature should precede the development of practice guidelines and serve as their foundation. This review must be well documented and easily available to those assessing or using a set of guidelines. It should describe all relevant aspects of the scientific research including (1) sponsors of the research, (2) investigators and their institutional affiliations, (3) research settings (for example, academic medical center or public outpatient clinic), (4) research populations, (5) methods (for example, randomized clinical trial), (6) limitations (for example, a research population limited to males when the condition or service under study is not), and (7) findings. The literature search method should also be described (for instance, MEDLARS), and the rules for including and excluding research should be explicitly noted (for example, whether unpublished materials or articles "in press" were used).

Altogether, the thoroughness of the review is a key step in developing valid guidelines, and documentation is a key requirement for later assessments of validity. The task, like those of estimating health outcomes and costs, may require the assistance of outside consultants or technical advisory panels. The qualifications of the individual or individuals responsible for the review should be described.

METHODS USED TO EVALUATE THE SCIENTIFIC LITERATURE

Methods for reviewing, summarizing, and evaluating the literature range from unarticulated and subjective—one person's unsupported synopsis, for instance—to highly formal, quantitative means of information synthesis and techniques of meta-analysis (Eddy, 1990b). The former approach is usually unsatisfactory for developing valid guidelines, and it is certainly no aid to those assessing guidelines independently. At a minimum, the factors considered in "weighing" or evaluating the evidence should be explicitly identified. For example, a reviewer could state that he or she weighed evidence from randomized clinical trials more heavily than evidence from case-control studies. An explicit rating of each entry in the literature used in the guidelines development process may be helpful but is not essential (Canadian Task Force on the Periodic Health Examination, 1979).

The more formal the analytic approach, the more valid the literature review (and hence the resulting guideline) can be expected to be. Formal approaches require that analysts guard against any application of quantitative and other systematic techniques that may disguise the limitations of incomplete or poor literature and thereby distort conclusions. The references to this chapter describe several formal approaches to evaluating evidence.

STRENGTH OF EVIDENCE

Inevitably, the evidence for some guidelines will be more abundant, consistent, clear, relevant, and methodologically rigorous than the evidence for others. Consequently, guidelines developers should provide some explicit description of the scientific certainty associated with a set of guidelines (Eddy, 1990a–e). The approach recently taken by the U.S. Preventive Services Task Force (1989) was to rank study designs; randomized controlled trials were ranked highest and expert opinion, lowest. However, this unidimensional scheme would rate a poorly executed randomized clinical trial more highly than a carefully done nonrandomized trial, a questionable result in the committee's view. More complex and statistically based techniques may be more accurate, but specific recommendations are beyond the scope of this committee.

One consequence of a thorough and expert assessment of the evidence may be a decision to defer the effort to develop guidelines for the condition or service in question because the evidence is weaker or less conclusive than expected when the effort was initiated. When it is imperative to go ahead with guidelines on a topic, the alternative is to rely more heavily on expert consensus. Even so, the experts may eventually agree that guidelines should be deferred for lack of either evidence or consensus.

USE OF EXPERT JUDGMENT

Expert or group judgment may come into play in guidelines development in two somewhat different but not incompatible ways. First, groups may be used to evaluate and rate scientific evidence with or without the support of quantitative methods such as meta-analysis. Second, group judgment may be used as the primary basis for a guideline when the scientific evidence is weak or nonexistent. Rather than have expert panels accept a consultant's or other party's review uncritically, the panels should conduct their own careful "review of the review" of the literature.

The methods used to arrive at group judgments must be carefully selected and well described (IOM, 1985). For example, if formal votes are taken, a secret, written ballot should be used, insofar as possible, and a record of the results of each round of voting should be maintained. Any departure from a policy of "one person-one vote" must be justified. If a panel member is absent from active group discussion of the guidelines, that absence should be noted. A recent IOM workshop on group judgment noted that more research needs to be done regarding the validity and reliability of judgments reached using different group judgment techniques (IOM, 1990f; Lomas, 1990).

STRENGTH OF EXPERT CONSENSUS

Expert groups will almost assuredly participate in the literature review and development of guidelines. The extent to which those experts agree on their findings and recommendations is important information. Thus, a set of guidelines should describe the strength and nature of the group consensus or agreement.

In some cases, the experts may strongly agree that clear evidence supports precise statements in a set of guidelines about the appropriateness or inappropriateness of a particular clinical practice. This agreement is powerful support for the validity of those statements. In other situations, experts may strongly agree that no clear evidence exists on which to base precise statements about appropriateness. This, too, is important information. In still other cases, the experts may disagree about what the evidence indicates and what statements about appropriateness are warranted (Park et al., 1986). These three quite different situations have different implications for guidelines developers and users.

The extent of agreement within an expert group should be reported in quantitative terms (for example, simple percentages describing levels of agreement or disagreement). When evidence or professional agreement is very strong, guidelines may be more confidently translated into criteria for evaluating practitioner performance.

INDEPENDENT REVIEW

In any endeavor involving expert panels and the subjective evaluation and interpretation of data, different groups may well arrive at different conclusions. Replication of guidelines development on the same clinical condition or technology is not likely to be feasible, affordable, or desirable (in terms of the opportunity costs involved). Therefore, at a minimum, some effort should be made to subject guidelines (including the relevant literature reviews) to review and criticism by professionals who are not involved in the original development process. These procedures should be described and the results summarized.

PRETESTING

Pretesting a set of guidelines on members of the intended user group (for example, practitioners or patients) using a real organization or a set of prototypical cases is desirable. (See also the discussions of reliability/reproducibility and clarity, below.) Description of methods, settings, and results of any pretests of the guidelines should be described. The Forum has been given authority to pretest guidelines, and the committee believes it should exercise that authority.

RELIABILITY/REPRODUCIBILITY

As conventionally used in a research context, reliability is linked to the measuring, diagnosing, or scoring of some phenomenon such as intelligence or bacterial infection.[5] In the context of guidelines, the committee uses the concept to refer to the ability of some method or process to produce consistent results across time or across users, or both. In strictly technical terms, levels of reliability dictate possible (achievable) levels of validity; that is, qualitative and quantitative instruments and tools cannot be valid if they are not reliable.

One kind of reliability is methodological. Ideally, if another group of qualified individuals using the same evidence, assumptions, and methods for guidelines development (for example, the same rules for literature review) were to develop guidelines, then they should produce essentially the same statements. In practice, such replications are almost unknown given the expense of the process,[6] but discussion of previous trials of the methodology (for different conditions) and any resulting revisions may be useful. Likewise, review of the guidelines by an outside panel can help in assessing reliability. (Recall that independent review is also important to an assessment of validity, a fact that underscores the link between reliability and validity.)

---

[5] The committee discussed how two common methodological concepts, *sensitivity* and *specificity*, applied to practice guidelines. For medical review and other evaluation criteria, these two related terms are fairly straightforward. Sensitivity and specificity refer, respectively, to a high "true positive rate" in detecting deficient or inappropriate care and a high "true negative rate" in passing over cases of adequate care. The concepts can be operationalized by requiring some evidence, drawn, for example, from pretesting of the review criteria on "prototype" cases or through pilot-testing in a specific organization. As described in Chapter 10 of the Medicare quality report, case-finding screens have often been found to be deficient on these two attributes. The committee concluded that these attributes need to be considered for evaluation instruments but do not add anything to the assessment of practice guidelines.

[6] One effort at replication has been undertaken by those involved with the RAND Corporation's work to develop appropriateness indicators (Chassin, 1990).

A second kind of reliability that is important for practice guidelines is clinical reliability. Practice guidelines are reliable if—given the same clinically relevant circumstances—the guidelines are interpreted and applied consistently by practitioners (or other appropriate parties). That is, the same practitioner, using the guidelines, makes the same basic clinical decision under the same circumstances from one time to the next, and different practitioners using the guidelines make the same decisions under the same circumstances. Pretesting of guidelines in actual delivery settings or on prototypical cases can help test this kind of reliability as well as contribute to assessments of validity.

For medical review criteria and other specific tools for evaluating health care actions or outcomes, the concept of reliability (or reproducibility) seems straightforward. Ideally, review criteria and other tools for evaluating performance should be pretested to provide evidence that they meet a specified level of reliability over time for the same user (test-retest reliability) and between users (interrater reliability). Review criteria often run into reliability problems when they use undefined terms—such as "frequent" or "serious" or "presence of comorbid conditions"—that different users may interpret quite differently. Thus, one tactic developers of guidelines and review criteria should use to maximize reliability is to avoid such terms unless precise definitions are provided.

CLINICAL APPLICABILITY

Because of the considerable resources and opportunity costs involved in developing practice guidelines, guidelines should be written to cover as inclusive a patient population as possible, consistent with knowledge about critical clinical and sociodemographic factors relevant for the condition or technology in question. For instance, a guideline should not be restricted to Medicare patients only through age 75 or through age 85 if evidence and expert judgment indicate that the clinical condition or the technology in question is pertinent to those over age 85.

This attribute requires that guidelines explicitly describe the population or populations to which statements apply. These populations may be defined in terms of diagnosis, pathophysiology, age, gender, race, social support systems, and other characteristics. The purpose of such a definition is to help physicians concentrate specific services on classes of patients that can benefit from those services and avoid such services for classes of patients for whom the services might do harm or produce no net benefit. Again, the relevant scientific literature needs to be cited or its absence noted.

CLINICAL FLEXIBILITY

Flexibility requires that a set of guidelines identify, where warranted, exceptions to their recommendations. The objective of this attribute is to allow necessary leeway for clinical judgment, patient preferences, and clinically relevant conditions of the delivery system (including necessary equipment and skilled personnel).[7]

Operationalizing this attribute may be difficult. In the committee's view, a fairly rigorous approach should be adopted, one that requires a set of guidelines to (1) list the major foreseeable exceptions and the rationale for such exceptions, (2) categorize generally the less foreseeable or highly idiosyncratic circumstances that may warrant exceptions, (3) describe the basic information to be provided to patients and the kinds of patient preferences that may be appropriately considered, and (4) indicate what data are needed to document exceptions based on clinical circumstances, patient preferences, or delivery system characteristics.

The role of patient preferences, whether considered in the context of daily clinical practice or in the context of developing guidelines, is a particularly complex issue. For example, there is much disagreement about the proper behavior for practitioners faced with preferences they believe are unreasonable or unacceptable (Brock and Wartman, 1990). Likewise, the balance between patient preferences and societal resources is the subject of intense debate.

A thorough treatment of this issue was not part of the committee's charge. However, in addition to recommending that patient interests be taken into account at several points in the process of developing guidelines, the committee makes two observations. First, patient preference for a service generally need not be acceded to when the service cannot be expected to provide any benefit or when it can be expected to produce a clear excess of harm over benefit. Second, when a mentally competent patient unreasonably wishes (in a practitioner's view) to forego treatment, the practitioner can try to persuade the patient to accept care but cannot, with rare exceptions, insist on treatment.

CLARITY

Clarity means that guidelines are written in unambiguous language. Their presentation is logically organized and easy to follow, and the use of abbreviations, symbols, and similar aids is consistent and well explained. Key terms and those subject to misinterpretation are defined. Vague clinical

---

[7] Clinical applicability and clinical flexibility could be grouped together as one attribute. Keeping them separate emphasizes the distinctions among the populations or settings that are covered by guidelines and those that are not so covered.

language, such as "severe bleeding," should be avoided in favor of more precise language, such as "a drop in hematocrit of more than 6 percent in less than eight hours." Similarly, guidelines must be specific about what populations and clinical circumstances are covered and what specific elements of care are appropriate, inappropriate, and (if relevant) equivocal, as those terms were defined earlier.

For practical reasons, assessments of language and modes of presentation may have to be largely subjective. Depending on the audience, somewhat different standards for assessing clarity may be needed. Materials for consumers might be subject to the "readability" measures that have been variously applied to regulations, consumer warranties, and similar materials. Materials for practitioners may be more technical but should not be burdened by needless jargon, awkward writing, or "unfriendly" software. Software itself may soon allow organizations to apply computer-based "style manuals" or "templates" to help standardize writing for different purposes (Frankel, 1990).

MULTIDISCIPLINARY PROCESS

One of the committee's strongest recommendations is that guidelines development include participation by representatives of key affected groups and disciplines.[8] The rationale for this position is threefold. First, multidisciplinary participation increases the probability that all relevant scientific evidence will be located and critically evaluated, thereby strengthening the scientific grounding, scope, and flexibility of the guidelines. Second, such participation increases the likelihood that practical problems with using guidelines will be identified and addressed, thus constructing a firmer foundation for successful application of the guidelines in real-world situations. Third, participation helps build a sense of involvement or "ownership" among different audiences for the guidelines, thereby improving the prospect for cooperation in implementing them. Figure 3-2 summarizes these rationales and other key issues in developing or assessing a participation strategy.

Among clinicians, multidisciplinary participation may call for the use of clinicians with and without full-time academic ties, for the inclusion of specialists and generalists, and for participation by relevant nonphysician practitioners. Optometrists, for instance, could well have an important role to play on panels to develop guidelines for cataract surgery. Experts in research and analytic methods also need to be represented on guidelines

---

[8] The term *multidisciplinary* is used broadly here rather than narrowly; it does not refer only to academic and professional disciplines.

WHY MULTIDISCIPLINARY PARTICIPATION IS NECESSARY

Strengthens scientific base of guidelines
Increases real-world utility
Creates sense of "ownership"
Expands foresight about conceptual and practical problems

WHO SHOULD PARTICIPATE

Clinicians
    Academic and nonacademic
    Specialists and generalists
    Physicians, nurses, and others as appropriate
Methodologists
    Experts in analyzing science bases
    Experts in group judgment methods
Nonclinician users
    Patients, potential patients, and families
    Payers and health plan sponsors
    Peer review and quality assurance experts
    Public policymakers

HOW PARTICIPATION MIGHT OCCUR

Membership on development panel
Testimony at public hearings
Review of draft guidelines
Focus groups
Consulting and contracting arrangements

WHEN PARTICIPATION MIGHT OCCUR

Early--setting the goals, determining the processes
Late--reviewing the results
Throughout--beginning to end and into implementation and evaluation

WHAT PARTICIPANTS MIGHT CONSIDER

Scope, quality, and evaluation of scientific evidence
Mode of presentation
Likely ease of application
Identification of user problems and needs

FIGURE 3-2 Multidisciplinary participation in guidelines development.

development panels; that is, methodological expertise should not be obtained only on a contractual basis or from specialized technical advisory panels.

User groups—in addition to clinicians—include health care administrators, members of peer review organizations, payers, and patients or consumers. If guidelines are expected to pertain to groups distinguished mainly by sociodemographic characteristics (for example, age or minority ethnic groups), special efforts are warranted to involve representatives of those groups at some early stage of development. Successful involvement of patients or consumers is a challenge that may require multiple strategies, as described below.

Documentation for this attribute will need to describe the parties involved, their credentials and potential biases, and the methods used to solicit their views and arrive at group judgments. The committee does not recommend, however, that the Forum develop detailed, rigid definitions of what constitutes a consumer or other participant category. (The often unproductive troubles such definitions created for federally funded health planning agencies were cited during the committee discussion.)

A frequent although not necessarily valid criticism of guidelines is that their content can be improperly manipulated by selecting group participants for their known opinions rather than on the basis of their expertise. The position taken here is that all participants in the guideline-setting process are likely to have personal opinions, biases, and preferences about the clinical problem or service at issue, and no amount of effort will expunge those factors. What is critical is that those factors be known and balanced insofar as possible.[9]

The committee discussed at some length the question of who should develop guidelines. Some members felt quite strongly that the Forum should not contract with medical specialty societies for guidelines development services. Others felt that establishing such a blanket prohibition was not the right approach. Instead, decisions should be based on a comparative assessment of potential developers' track records and capacities. These capabilities include, for example, related work that the groups or individual participants have already done, existing documentation of participants' credentials and biases, and the methods and evidence with which they have experience. Although the committee did not reach a specific consensus that the Forum should completely exclude specialty societies as potential direct contractors or subcontractors, the agency should be sensitive to the credibility concerns raised by this question. Physician organizations in any case should be extensively consulted by developers of guidelines, involved in reviewing draft guidelines, and used to help disseminate guidelines.

Another debate arose during the committee's meetings over the question of who should chair a guidelines development group. Again, some

---

[9] The procedures of the National Academy of Sciences might serve as a model for the panel selection process. These procedures require that members of study committees submit bias statements and that an official of the Academy lead each committee through a member-by-member discussion of possible biases. Major funders of a study cannot be represented on a study committee, and every committee report must be reviewed by a panel of outside experts under the oversight of the National Research Council.

felt that a specialist user of a particular technology (for example, a cardiac surgeon who performs coronary artery bypass surgery) should never chair a group developing guidelines on the use of that technology. Others felt that exceptions to the general principle might sometimes be warranted. There was considerable agreement that a physician should chair the development of any clinical practice guidelines. Again, explicit attention to questions of bias is essential.

Participation by affected groups in the process of guidelines development can be achieved in several ways. The strongest form of participation is membership on the panel charged with developing guidelines, but the benefits of this approach have to be balanced against the practical management problems created by too large a panel. Participation may also be achieved through mechanisms other than the panel—for example, public hearings, circulation of draft guidelines for review and comment by a wide variety of groups, and contracts with particular interests for specific analyses. Focus groups and pretests may uncover confusing language or highlight the "hassle factor" associated with draft guidelines and allow practitioners or patients to suggest more acceptable alternatives.

Different types of guidelines are likely to require different mechanisms for participation, and the benefits of participation need to be balanced against resource limitations and other constraints. Therefore, this report stresses the principle and value of participation rather than the specific vehicles. Creativity and experimentation should, in fact, be encouraged.

SCHEDULED REVIEW

Clinical evidence and judgment are not static. Therefore, guidelines should designate a review date to determine whether they should be updated or, potentially, withdrawn. In a clinical area where technologies are changing rapidly and new research findings can be expected to accumulate quickly, a relatively short timetable may be appropriate. More stable clinical areas may permit a longer period before scheduled review. In every case, however, a guideline should contain a specific review date or time frame for review (for example, within three years of initial publication). The greater the amount of change in a clinical area, the more the revision process will resemble the initial development process in scope, cost, and intensity.

Follow-up on review schedules is part of the implementation process (see Chapter 4) as is determination of whether review is needed before the scheduled date. Unscheduled revisions may be prompted by major new clinical evidence or by emerging or disintegrating professional consensus. To oversee both scheduled and unscheduled reviews, an organization responsible for the development of multiple sets of guidelines should subject

TABLE 3-2 Provisional Documentation Checklist for Practice Guidelines

Attribute	Item
Validity	Projected health outcomes if guidelines are followed. Information required to evaluate outcomes.
	Projected costs if guidelines are followed. Information required to evaluate costs.
	Description of data, methods, and assumptions used to make projections.
	Explicit description of the relationship between the scientific evidence and the guidelines *and* explanations for any differences between the guidelines and the evidence. Explanations for any important differences between the guidelines in question and those developed by others.
	Thorough literature review describing scientific research including sponsors, settings, methodologies, findings, and qualifications.
	Description of methodology for evaluating the scientific literature and the results.
	Explicit assessment of the quality, consistency, clarity, and strength of the scientific evidence.
	Description of methodology for using expert or group judgment as a basis for evaluating scientific evidence or, in the absence of evidence, reaching a consensus based on expert opinion.
	Explicit description of the strength of expert consensus.
	Description of procedures, participants, and findings of review by experts and others not involved in the original development process.
	Description of methods, settings, and results of any pretests of the guidelines.
Reliability/ reproducibility	Description of methods and results of testing (1) the reliability of the development method and (2) the reproducibility of the clinical decisions reached by users of the guidelines.

all of its guidelines to some kind of yearly examination to flag particular guidelines for either scheduled or unscheduled review. As described in the next chapter, the mechanisms for disseminating and administering guidelines need to provide for guidelines updating or withdrawal.

DOCUMENTATION

For the purposes of emphasis, the committee lists documentation as a separate attribute even though it has already been referred to repeatedly in the discussion of other attributes. As a practical matter, a documentation checklist, such as the preliminary version presented in Table 3-2, may be helpful for contractors and review panels.

TABLE 3-2 continued

Attribute	Item
Clinical applicability	Specification by age, sex, race, clinical diagnosis, and other factors of the populations to which a set of guidelines apply. Description and analysis of the scientific literature or expert consensus that forms the basis for statements about the age, sex, and other factors of the populations to which a set of guidelines apply.
Clinical flexibility	Description and analysis of the scientific literature or expert consensus that forms the basis for statements about major foreseeable exceptions to application of the guidelines. Listing of the basic information to be provided to patients and the kinds of patient preferences that may be appropriately considered. Listing of the data needed to document exceptions based on clinical circumstances, patient preferences, or delivery system characteristics.
Clarity	Methods and results of any testing of readability, logic, or understanding.
Multidisciplinary process	Description of the parties involved in developing the guidelines, their credentials and interests, and the methods used to solicit their views or to arrive at group judgments. Description of the procedures used to subject guidelines to review and criticism by experts not involved in the original development process, with summary of results.
Scheduled review	Timetable and method for the scheduled review. Description of the basis for arriving at the timetable or specific date.

CONCLUSION

This chapter has proposed eight attributes of practice guidelines that the Forum should employ in advising its contractors and expert panels and in assessing the quality of the guidelines it receives. The attributes are validity, reliability (reproducibility), clinical applicability, clinical flexibility, clarity, multidisciplinary process, scheduled review, and documentation. Definitions of these terms and some examples that may aid in their operationalization are also given. Operationalization, that is, turning these eight concepts into a practical instrument for the Forum to use in prospectively assessing guidelines, is one task in a broader project that the IOM is currently conducting (Appendix C).

Several issues about guidelines development need to be kept in mind as the Forum proceeds. First, neither existing guidelines nor those likely to be developed by the agency in the foreseeable future will "score well" on all eight properties simultaneously; indeed, near-perfect scores may always lie in the realm of aspiration rather than attainment. Second, a balance needs to be maintained between an ideal process and a feasible one. For example, this committee, and others, could design a very meticulous process to take into account the views of all interested groups. At some level, that process would consume more resources—in time, professional input, and money—than the outputs would warrant. That is, it would be too slow, too cumbersome to administer, and too costly to meet the needs of providers, third-party payers, or patients. It undoubtedly would not conform to the congressional deadlines of OBRA 89.

The third point to stress is that guidelines development must be an evolutionary process, especially at the national (or federal) level. There is no proven "right way" to conduct this endeavor, even if there clearly are some "better ways." Guidelines that satisfactorily reflect the eight attributes proposed here may not be products of an ideal process, but in the committee's view they will be defensible.

Two other themes should be reiterated: the need for credibility among practitioners, patients, payers, and policymakers, and the need for accountability. The entire practice guidelines enterprise will not fulfill its promise (and certainly the federal program will not) if the products lack solid scientific grounding and widespread understanding and support from the provider and patient communities. The significance accorded such attributes as validity and reliability, clarity, multidisciplinary approach, and documentation reflects the committee's concerns with these needs. Although in the first instance the themes of credibility and accountability apply to the procedures followed in guidelines development, they also carry through to the procedures of implementation and evaluation, which are the subjects of the next chapter.

REFERENCES

American College of Physicians. *Clinical Efficacy Assessment Project: Procedural Manual.* Philadelphia, Pa.: 1986.
American Medical Association. *Attributes to Guide the Development of Practice Parameters.* Chicago, Ill.: American Medical Association, 1990a.
American Medical Association. Preliminary Worksheet for the Evaluation of Practice Parameters. Draft of ad hoc review panel. Chicago, Illinois, May 1990b.
Canadian Task Force on the Periodic Health Examination. *Canadian Medical Association Journal* 121:1193–1254, 1979.
Battista, R., and Fletcher, S. Making Recommendations on Preventive Practices: Methodological Issues. *American Journal of Preventive Medicine* 4:53–67, 1988 (Supplement).
Brock, D., and Wartman, S. When Competent Patients Make Irrational Choices. *New England Journal of Medicine* 322:1595–1599, 1990.
Chassin, Mark. Presentation to the IOM Committee to Advise the Public Health Service on Practice Guidelines. Washington, D.C., April 2, 1990.
Eddy, D. Comparing Benefits and Harms: The Balance Sheet. *Journal of the American Medical Association* 263:2493–2505, 1990a.

Eddy, D. Guidelines for Policy Statements: The Explicit Approach. *Journal of the American Medical Association* 263:2239–2240, 1990b.

Eddy, D. Practice Policies—Guidelines for Methods. *Journal of the American Medical Association* 263:1839–1841, 1990c.

Eddy, D. Practice Policies—What Are They? *Journal of the American Medical Association* 263:877–880, 1990d.

Eddy, D. Practice Policies—Where Do They Come From? *Journal of the American Medical Association* 263:1265–1275, 1990e.

Eddy, D. Designing a Practice Policy: Standards, Guidelines, and Options. *Journal of the American Medical Association*, forthcoming (a).

Eddy, D. *A Manual for Assessing Health Practices and Designing Practice Policies.* American College of Physicians, forthcoming (b).

Eddy, D., and Billings, J. The Quality of Medical Evidence and Medical Practice. Paper prepared for the National Leadership Commission on Health, Washington, D.C., 1988.

Fink, A., Kosecoff, J., Chassin, M., et al. Consensus Methods: Characteristics and Guidelines for Use. *American Journal of Public Health* 74:979–983, 1984.

Frankel, S. Hello, Mr. Chips: PCs Learn English. *Washington Post*, April 29, 1990, p. D3.

Gottlieb, L., Margolis, C., and Schoenbaum, S. Clinical Practice Guidelines at an HMO: Development and Implementation in a Quality Improvement Model. *Quality Review Bulletin* 16:80–86, 1990.

Institute of Medicine. Effects of Clinical Evaluation on the Diffusion of Medical Technology. Chapter 4 in *Assessing Medical Technologies.* Washington, D.C.: National Academy Press, 1985.

Institute of Medicine. *Acute Myocardial Infarction: Setting Priorities for Effectiveness Research.* Washington, D.C.: National Academy Press, 1990a.

Institute of Medicine. *Breast Cancer: Setting Priorities for Effectiveness Research.* Washington, D.C.: National Academy Press, 1990b.

Institute of Medicine. *Hip Fracture: Setting Priorities for Effectiveness Research.* Washington, D.C.: National Academy Press, 1990c.

Institute of Medicine. *Medicare: A Strategy for Quality Assurance,* Lohr, K., ed. Washington, D.C.: National Academy Press, 1990d.

Institute of Medicine. *National Priorities for the Assessment of Clinical Conditions and Medical Technologies,* Lara, M., and Goodman, C., eds. Washington, D.C.: National Academy Press, 1990e.

Institute of Medicine. Workshop to Improve Group Judgment for Medical Practice and Technology Assessment, Washington, D.C., May 15–16, 1990f.

Lomas, J. Words Without Action? The Production, Dissemination and Impact of Consensus Recommendations. Draft paper (dated May 1990) prepared for the *Annual Review of Public Health*, Vol. 12, Omenn, G., ed. Palo Alto, Calif., forthcoming.

Mulley, A. Presentation to the Workshop to Improve Group Judgment for Medical Practice and Technology Assessment, Washington, D.C., May 15, 1990.

National Research Council. *Improving Risk Communication.* Washington, D.C.: National Academy Press, 1989.

Park, R., Fink, A., Brook, R., et al. *Physician Ratings of Appropriate Indications for Six Medical and Surgical Procedures.* R-3280-CWF/HF/PMT/RWJ. Santa Monica, Calif.: The RAND Corporation, 1986. See also the same authors and same title in the *American Journal of Public Health* 76:766–772, 1986.

U.S. Preventive Services Task Force. *Guide to Clinical Preventive Services: An Assessment of the Effectiveness of 169 Interventions.* Baltimore, Md.: Williams & Wilkins, 1989.

4

Implementation and Evaluation

The separation of policy design from implementation is fatal.

Pressman and Wildavsky, *Implementation*

The primary charge to the study committee was to advise AHCPR and the Forum about definitions and attributes of guidelines with an emphasis on the agency's near-term responsibilities. Therefore, the committee was quite selective in its attention to implementation and evaluation matters. The major proposition here is that implementation and evaluation strategies should reinforce the credibility, validity, clarity, and other attributes of good guidelines identified in Chapter 3.

The committee's examination of implementation and evaluation issues began with six basic propositions.

- First, guidelines are not self-implementing.
- Second, the effectiveness of guidelines in reaching their intended objectives cannot be assumed but must be tested.
- Third, attention to implementation and evaluation issues should be built into the processes of guidelines development rather than dealt with sequentially.
- Fourth, many parties must contribute if guidelines are to be successfully implemented and evaluated.
- Fifth, the eventual revision or redesign of guidelines and their

implementation processes needs to be anticipated as guidelines are first disseminated, used, and evaluated.

- Sixth, implementation processes will not be static but will evolve as better methods are identified and less successful approaches are discarded. Such evolution may complicate evaluation.

The rest of this chapter emphasizes practice guidelines and makes only occasional comments about medical review criteria, performance measures, and standards of quality. Implementation is discussed first, followed by a shorter section on evaluation.

TYPES OF IMPLEMENTATION

Implementation refers to the concrete activities and interventions undertaken to turn policy objectives into desired outcomes (Pressman and Wildavsky, 1973). In the context of this report, these activities are viewed as a set of partly coordinated, partly disjointed steps or activities that include formatting, disseminating, applying, and revising or updating guidelines.

Two overlapping but distinct implementation tasks can be distinguished. One is implementing the public program established by OBRA 89. The other is implementing the practice guidelines themselves.

PROGRAM IMPLEMENTATION

OBRA 89 gives primary responsibility for establishing a program to develop and promote practice guidelines to the Department of Health and Human Services (DHHS) through AHCPR and its Forum. Necessary steps for implementing this program include hiring staff, developing a program agenda, establishing an advisory council, letting contracts, convening expert panels, and generally establishing and administering a broad, ongoing federal program.[1] The IOM committee's advice about definitions and attributes of guidelines is intended to assist the agency with two aspects of program implementation: working with expert panels and assessing the results.

Congress provided for an Advisory Council for Health Care Policy, Research, and Evaluation to advise the Secretary and the administrator of AHCPR on a broad array of activities. Council advice on the development of guidelines and the conduct of outcomes research must be handled by a special Subcouncil on Outcomes and Guidelines. Neither the Council

---

[1] Private organizations, such as the American College of Physicians (ACP) and others that develop guidelines, face program implementation tasks that are similar in many respects to those faced by the Forum (ACP, 1986). The same statement applies to guidelines implementation.

nor the Subcouncil has explicit responsibilities for program oversight, and it remains to be seen what their specific roles will be with respect to the program.

The Forum can underscore its intent to examine critically and improve its program and products in at least three ways. First, it should ask its expert panels for feedback on the strengths and weaknesses of the procedures followed. Second, the Forum should pretest (or arrange for the pretesting of) all guidelines developed under its aegis. This can be done on a pilot basis in a real delivery setting, on a set of prototypical cases, or by both methods, but it needs to be done. Third, the Forum should try to evaluate the effectiveness of intermediate actions (for example, formatting, dissemination, incentives) that are necessary if guidelines are to have their intended effects on health practices, outcomes, and costs. Each of these steps can be part of a learning process for the Forum and others.

GUIDELINES IMPLEMENTATION

The second implementation task—the focus of this chapter—involves taking a set of practice guidelines, once they have been developed, into the actual world of health care delivery. It is in such a sphere that guidelines will prove themselves as effective or ineffective interventions.

Government Responsibilities for Implementing Guidelines

OBRA 89 outlined certain responsibilities for AHCPR and the Forum that relate directly to the implementation of practice guidelines. The Forum was specifically directed to concern itself with formats of guidelines (for medical educators, consumers, practitioners, and medical review organizations) and with disseminating and otherwise making guidelines available. More generally, the legislation requires that the Secretary of Health and Human Services "provide for the use of [the initial set of] guidelines. . .to improve the quality, effectiveness, and appropriateness of care provided under Title XVIII." This and other legislative language implies the involvement of other federal agencies such as the Health Care Financing Administration (HCFA) and the National Library of Medicine (NLM). Although nothing is said about the role of government as a direct provider of health care services, the health care systems administered by the Department of Defense, the Department of Veterans Affairs, and the Public Health Service clearly allow a government role in implementing guidelines in health care settings.

Roles of Other Organizations in Implementing Guidelines

Absent further legislation or regulations to the contrary, the federal government will not be the major actor in implementing guidelines. Rather, an array of private individuals and organizations will be the crucial participants in every stage of implementation. OBRA 89 refers explicitly to the involvement of provider and consumer organizations, medical educators, peer review organizations, and accrediting bodies in the dissemination of guidelines, but dissemination is only one step in assuring that guidelines are applied by clinicians and patients to improve health care outcomes. What goes on in delivery settings such as hospitals, physician offices, and nursing homes is the key to successful implementation. The foundation for such success, however, starts much earlier during the process of guidelines development.

LINKS BETWEEN DEVELOPMENT AND IMPLEMENTATION STAGES

In discussing the attributes of good guidelines in Chapter 3, the committee has underscored the link between development and implementation in several ways, including the following examples.

1. The credibility of the development process, the participants, and the scientific grounding of guidelines must be clear to intended users.

2. A truly multidisciplinary approach to guidelines development will facilitate acceptance and use of guidelines by members of the groups represented and by other, secondary groups.

3. Guidelines should be specific, comprehensive, and flexible enough to be useful in the varied settings and circumstances of everyday medical practice and in the evolving programs to assess the appropriateness of care provided in these settings.

4. Guidelines language, logic, and symbols should be easy to follow and unambiguous, so that movement from guidelines to educational tools, review criteria, or other instruments is unimpeded.

5. Pretesting is highly useful; it can be done on a pilot basis in a real delivery setting, on a set of prototypical cases, or by both methods.

6. The guidelines should specify what information about the clinical problem, the patient's circumstances and preferences, and the delivery setting should be recorded to permit later evaluation of the appropriateness of care (judged against criteria generated from the guidelines).

Developers of guidelines need to be cognizant of the practical realities involved in translating guidelines into medical review criteria and applying those criteria for quality assurance and other purposes. Such foresight is important whether the processes of guidelines and criteria development are undertaken by the same or different bodies. Of the precepts listed above, those relating to clinical specificity, clarity, and data recording can be particularly useful in assisting the move from guidelines for practitioners to criteria for assessing health care practice.

To say that implementation needs to be considered as guidelines are developed is not to imply that every step and detail can be or needs to be foreseen. That kind of foresight is impossible. Moreover, just as there is no "one best way" yet identified or demonstrated to develop guidelines, neither is there one best way to implement them. Pluralism in both phases is likely to be the norm for the present.

PLANNING FOR IMPLEMENTATION

Clearly, successful implementation will depend on many factors in addition to the quality and credibility of the guidelines and their design process. Among those factors are (1) the funding for dissemination and other implementation activities; (2) the incentives and supports for the guidelines to be used by practitioners, health plans, and others; (3) the accessibility, scope, accuracy, and timeliness of a variety of intra- and interorganizational information systems; and (4) the ability of multiple parties to plan and execute the various steps needed to implement guidelines.

Compared with the processes of designing guidelines, the processes of implementation tend to be more diffuse. The time horizon extends beyond the near future, the number of involved parties multiplies, local circumstances become more important, responsibilities blur, and actions become more difficult to track. These conditions make it more difficult to specify attributes of an implementation process in the way Chapter 3 specified the attributes of guidelines. Nonetheless, some of the factors that need to be considered in making implementation decisions can be articulated as noted below.

• The particular *objectives* to be served by the implementation process. Examples: rapidly informing practitioners of new guidelines that depart significantly from previous guidelines; providing immediate and continuously available assistance to practitioners as they diagnose or treat particular patients; educating consumers about the use of screening services (Avorn and Somerai, 1983; Lundberg, 1989; Somerai and Avorn, 1990).

• The expected *effectiveness* of alternative strategies in achieving the objectives in question. Examples: the impact of direct mail notification compared with publication in a journal; the accessibility of an interactive computer system versus printed instructions (Jacoby and Clarke, 1986).

• The *cost* of alternative strategies in relation to the expected benefit and the *available resources*. Examples: the cost of a press conference versus a direct mailing; the cost of a desktop compendium of guidelines versus a computer-based expert system.

- The *demands* made on target users by different alternatives. Example: the learning required for user-friendly versus non-user-friendly computer software.
- The *manageability* of the tasks for administrators or others responsible for implementing a decision. Example: setting up a system of financial incentives compared with setting up an information feedback system.

Selecting the particular elements of an implementation plan requires assessment of these and other variables. Inevitably, trade-offs will be required among some factors such as expected effectiveness and cost or manageability.

ELEMENTS OF IMPLEMENTATION

In this context, implementation has four main aspects: formatting, disseminating, applying, and updating. These categorizations partly reflect OBRA 89 language. As a result, the discussion below uses some rather narrow definitions that should not be applied rigidly.

FORMATTING

Formatting refers to the presentation of guidelines in physical arrangements or media that can be readily understood by a designated set of users, for example, practitioners or patients. Different formats may be appropriate for different users and settings, for different means of dissemination, and for different types of guidelines.

To the extent that the Forum asks developers of guidelines to assume responsibility for formatting, this task is less an implementation step than an initial design step. However, because formatting is so closely related to dissemination and application and because the responsibility for formatting is likely to be shared between developers and implementers, it is discussed here rather than in Chapter 3. In any case, the Forum will need to prepare some instructions on layout and sequencing of material for its panels and contractors.

Formatting here emphasizes *physical layout and logic*; dissemination, on the other hand, focuses on the *roles of different parties and media* in getting information to different groups. Thus, for example, the physical properties and logic of documents or computer software are formatting issues, but decisions about how much and when to rely on written documents versus computer software are dissemination issues.

Although the committee examined an extensive set of examples of printed formats of practice guidelines and related materials,[2] it was not able to review any empirical evidence on the effectiveness of different formats. Thus, the committee considered it inappropriate to recommend specific formats to the Forum. The materials examined—viewed in the context of the attributes described in Chapter 3—did lead to several subjective judgments about simple features that distinguish better formats from inferior formats. These features include (1) one- or two-page summaries of key recommendations and rationales; (2) readily located descriptions of the development process, assumptions, objectives, methods, definitions, and participants; (3) selective use of boldface, subheadings, and other highlighting techniques; (4) attractive typefaces and graphic aids; and (5) uncrowded layouts (for example, pages with ample margins and other "white space"). An index to major elements of the guidelines and a glossary of key terms and symbols might also be considered. In addition, a prominent listing of sources for additional information on the guidelines (or for related guidelines) may be a useful adjunct.

More generally, regardless of whether formatting is treated as a design step or an implementation step, the attributes of guidelines related to credibility and accountability should be reinforced by the physical layout. For example, the user should quickly "see" that the guidelines emerged from a multidisciplinary process strongly grounded in scientific evidence and analysis including projections of health and cost outcomes.

The attributes of clarity and reliability/reproducibility discussed in the preceding chapter are central. Logical presentation, precise terminology, clear and consistent use of words, phrases, and symbols, and similar properties must be features of acceptable formats so that the guidelines are correctly and consistently understood. Likewise, users should be able to locate easily the descriptions of the populations covered by the guidelines and the identified exceptions. If guidelines describe patient care documentation that practitioners should provide, a prominent summary or checklist of such documentation needs is desirable.

How the attributes of good guidelines can best be reinforced by formatting choices will differ depending on whether the medium of dissemination is, for example, a journal article or a computerized decision support system.

---

[2] The majority of the materials reviewed by the committee pertained to clinicians (mainly physicians but also nurses) and included algorithms to guide patient management; statements about the appropriateness (or inappropriateness) of specific preventive, diagnostic, or therapeutic procedures; information about prescription drugs from the *Physician's Desk Reference* (1990); the AMA Diagnostic and Therapeutic Technology Assessment (DATTA) Evaluation series; the online cancer protocols of Physician Data Query (PDQ); and up-to-date information from *Scientific American Medicine* (Rubenstein and Federman, 1989). The committee also considered materials aimed at patients, such as the algorithms developed by Vickery and Fries (1986) to guide decisionmaking by patients at home, and other materials focused more exclusively on medical education.

Again, trade-offs are inevitable. For instance, "desktop" compendiums of guidelines will involve trade-offs among appealing formats, accessible language, and ready availability of many different guidelines.

The importance of appealing, accessible presentations of guidelines for practitioners and patients is often underestimated (and the development of such presentations underfunded). Presentation is not merely a frill but an aspect of guidelines implementation that requires serious attention. Nonetheless, as for every other step described in this report, the development of effective formats will have to compete with other priorities and will involve learning over time about what works better. To help that learning occur, the Forum should allocate some of its limited resources (or seek assistance from outside sources) to evaluate the effectiveness of alternative formats and media. In the short term, the Forum should encourage its expert panels or contractors to offer suggestions about layout and to produce, in addition to any format required by the Forum, an alternative document if the group judges that alternative to be superior.

DISSEMINATION

Dissemination as it is used here means getting guidelines to the intended users, particularly when they are initially published, adopted, or updated. Dissemination may occur in several phases or waves (Kaluzny, 1990). The first step comes when the government or other sponsor of guidelines development begins to publicize the development of a new set of guidelines. Generally, this publicity involves enlisting the aid of other organizations such as medical specialty societies. Second, even without the sponsor's intervention, other parties—including the news media, computer information systems, professional colleagues, and workplace health promotion programs—may help spread information. As hospitals, HMOs, and other organizations decide that the guidelines should be adopted for internal use, they will communicate them to physicians, nurses, and others.

Because many organizations are developing guidelines, the AHCPR and its Forum are considering the need for a clearinghouse function and their relation to it. The committee did not consider this role in depth but notes that the quality of guidelines needs to be considered in any clearinghouse activity. Wider dissemination of poor guidelines is not in the public interest.

As described below, the focus of dissemination is on creating awareness and general understanding. Providing the practitioner with ongoing, routine access to information in an actual delivery setting is treated here as an administrative issue (as described in the next section).

Legislatively and practically, the Forum's dissemination strategies will rely heavily on the capacities and preferences of private or quasi-public groups such as medical organizations, consumer groups, and peer review organizations (PROs). As a consequence, no matter how cooperative these organizations are, many specific dissemination decisions will lie beyond the substantial influence of the Forum. Recognizing this, the committee offers only a few observations that may help the Forum and others in thinking about dissemination and its limits.

The themes of credibility and accountability are relevant to decisions about dissemination. For example, using the journals, conferences, and other communication vehicles of medical specialty groups is more likely to lend credibility to the guidelines than using a Forum press release or a PRO newsletter. The former approach may also provide more opportunity for "full disclosure," thereby enhancing the accountability of the process. Personal presentations by those involved in developing guidelines may likewise have more impact than publicity statements, but such presentations imply the availability of a cadre of well-prepared presenters.

Trade-offs are inevitable. For example, a press release may be the quickest vehicle for bringing high-priority guidelines[3] to public and practitioner attention, but this timeliness typically comes at the loss (at least in the short run) of important information for different parties and the loss of some credibility with practitioners. PRO and carrier announcements are likely to be a swift mechanism for bringing Medicare-relevant guidelines to the attention of the medical community, but they are far less likely to reach the general public.

The credibility and completeness of the information made available through on-line computer data bases (for example, MEDLARS) will depend on a variety of specific decisions about content, the extent of material to be available, retrieval rules, and development and access costs. Some evidence on the NLM's Physician Data Query (PDQ) suggests that patients are as likely as physicians to use that computerized information system, a finding that, if true of other, similar data bases, could raise some questions about how to target and present information (L. Blankenbaker, comments during an AHCPR methodology workshop, Rockville, Md., May 30, 1990).

Dissemination of guidelines by PROs in the form of review criteria may be particularly helpful in focusing practitioner attention on the groups covered by the guidelines and on the exceptions. The PRO path of dissemination may, in turn, create an early feedback loop for updating the guidelines or criteria when important omissions are identified. For

---

[3] Such guidelines include those involving a dramatic change from previous guidelines or those involving information that, if quickly applied, could significantly affect mortality or morbidity (Moldover, 1990; Steinbrook and Lo, 1990; "Word of Spinal-Injury Drug Not Getting Out," *Washington Post*, 1990).

these reasons, early and formal involvement of the PRO community in the guidelines development process seems highly desirable.

The development of computer-based expert systems may also include feedback provisions. More important, the use of such systems is likely to enhance the reliability and validity of clinical decisionmaking.

APPLICATION AND ADMINISTRATION OF GUIDELINES

Administering practice guidelines refers to the practical activities required for users to apply the guidelines in making specific decisions about appropriate health care for particular patients or classes of patients. As noted earlier, it is unrealistic to expect the developers of guidelines to anticipate all the contingencies that different users of guidelines will routinely face. Some adaptation is an inevitable and frequently desirable feature of guidelines application.

The primary individual appliers of practice guidelines are, in the short run, likely to be physicians, nurses, or other clinicians whose services come within the scope of a particular set of guidelines. The greater the role of the patient in making a health care decision, the more the patient will be a primary individual user of guidelines. The primary organizational appliers of practice guidelines will be health care providers including hospitals, nursing homes, group practices, and public clinics.

The primary users of medical review criteria, standards of quality, and performance measures should be, first, health care providers in their internal review and monitoring programs and, second, external quality review programs, health benefit plans, and claims payers. Placing health care providers first as users of these instruments reinforces the call of the recent IOM report on quality assurance for Medicare (1990) for increased emphasis on professional self-review, outcomes assessment, and information feedback.

OBRA 89 holds AHCPR and its Forum accountable for administering a government program, *not* for administering guidelines in a health care setting. The Forum and other government agencies may, however, support the application of guidelines at the practice level by funding the development of computer-based medical decision systems and similar activities. HCFA and its contractors are likely to administer medical review criteria for such purposes as preprocedure review, quality assurance, and claims administration for Medicare.

Other agencies of the federal government, such as the Department of Veterans Affairs, the Department of Defense, and the Indian Health Service, presumably can have a more direct role in using guidelines, performance measures, medical review criteria, and standards of quality in hospitals, clinics, and similar delivery settings. Conceivably, these agencies could be laboratories for testing guidelines and alternative ways of implementing them.

Provider Organizations

Administrative processes to support the application of guidelines will vary depending on an organization's purposes, structure, and resources. For example, staff-model HMOs, independent practice associations (IPAs), and public clinics may differ in how they integrate the use of guidelines with ongoing organizational programs such as staff education and patient outreach. The type of targeted mammography screening guidelines and programs that a staff-model HMO with a stable membership can manage (Field, 1990) would seem to be of questionable feasibility for a clinic serving migrant workers. Similarly, organizations with more resources (for example, libraries, video centers, telephone hotlines, personal computers, and access to local and national computer information systems) will be able to facilitate the use of guidelines in ways that are out of reach for less resource-rich organizations. Some organizations may want to establish formal programs to encourage adherence to guidelines. Such programs might include (1) preparation of *standard operating procedures* for staff (for example, for checking anesthesia equipment), (2) *contracting* with practitioners based on their acceptance of selected guidelines, or (3) *periodic feedback* on how an individual practitioner's behavior compares with both peer practices and specific guidelines. These mechanisms can reinforce guidelines along several dimensions including validity, reliability, and credibility.

Review Organizations

Medical review criteria and other evaluation instruments, if properly developed and sensitively applied, can create incentives for adherence to practice guidelines. If poorly developed and insensitively applied, they can undermine support for practice guidelines. Fortunately, the processes of translating guidelines into review criteria and then applying them provide one opportunity for early identification and correction of omissions. The Forum may want to consider establishing early contact with the peer review and quality assurance communities to help ensure the best possible movement of guidelines into these applications. No one, however, should underestimate the challenges this movement entails.

As discussed in Chapter 3, this committee's charge did not include recommendations on principles and techniques for translating guidelines into practice evaluation instruments. However, because review procedures have the potential either to support or undermine guidelines, the committee wishes to set forth several principles for structuring and managing the review process based on earlier IOM reports on utilization management (1989) and quality assurance (1990).

1.   Consistent with the recommendations of the IOM report on private-sector utilization management, review criteria should be *public* with respect to their content and their development process. (This does not require that software and other administrative tools be public.)

2.   When criteria are used to assess quality of care, deny payment for specific services, or take similar steps, an *appeals process* needs to be provided. This process must be clearly described to patients and practitioners and be free from unreasonable complexity, delay, or other barriers.

3.   Review organizations should make their review activities as *manageable* and *nonintrusive* as possible for both patients and practitioners. These organizations are one contributor to the growing "hassle factor" in medical care.

4.   Insofar as possible, review organizations should provide *constructive* information and feedback to physicians aimed at improving practice rather than punishing missteps.

The Forum will need to work with provider groups, HCFA, the PROs, and other organizations to encourage careful development and application of review criteria and other practice evaluation tools. These are not simple or unimportant tasks.

Other Organizations

Organizations involved with medical informatics and education clearly have a role to play in the dissemination and administration of practice guidelines. Many researchers, practitioners, and institutions are now involved in developing prototype expert systems and other computer support for information retrieval, decisionmaking, and monitoring (Shortliffe, 1987; Greenes and Shortliffe, 1990; Williamson et al., 1989). The relative utility of different approaches, for example, comprehensive nationwide systems (such as PDQ) versus institution- or service-specific systems, should be evaluated. Intended users of information systems may not, in fact, find them useful.

The widespread use of information and decision support systems will, however, probably require extensive involvement of commercial enterprises with the capital and expertise to develop, market, and maintain generally usable software, consulting services, and so forth. AHCPR may want to give early consideration to its stance on such commercial developments as they pertain to the guidelines emerging from expert panels.

In another area, the medical specialty boards may provide a powerful incentive for the understanding and use of guidelines. For instance, information and practice behaviors relating to guidelines can be built into both certification and periodic recertification procedures. Several medical specialty boards are considering the role of practice guidelines in the practice assessments they undertake or plan to undertake as part of their certification activities. Although steps such as these carry the application and administration of practice guidelines far from the immediate practical concerns of AHCPR, the potential importance of many disparate national and local organizations in the broader scheme of guidelines implementation should not be ignored.

UPDATING AND REVISING

In discussing attributes of guidelines, the committee proposed that developers of practice guidelines specify a date or timetable for a review to determine whether revisions to the guidelines are warranted. Reviews could come earlier than scheduled if there were indications of new clinical evidence or changing professional consensus. The credibility and accountability of this process is as essential as that of the initial process of developing guidelines.

The Forum thus needs to establish a follow-up mechanism to see that scheduled review occurs and that unscheduled reviews are initiated when necessary. In addition, the Forum should specify procedures for determining whether revisions are actually warranted and, if so, how those revisions will take place. The first step could be undertaken by AHCPR staff, by contractors, or by an advisory panel. It could include, in addition to the review of new clinical literature or evaluations of the guidelines' impact, a request for comments published in the *Federal Register*. The second step could involve convening new expert panels to make revisions consistent with the attributes specified in the previous chapter.

To the extent that parties outside the government are developing similar or related guidelines, the Forum may also want to support a separate effort to review such "outside" guidelines as a means of informing its own priorities and processes. This activity could be incorporated into a clearinghouse function.

The committee was concerned during its deliberations with the problem of inconsistent guidelines. By determining how the guidelines sponsored by AHCPR and those developed by others conform to each other and then investigating the reasons for inconsistencies, the agency may identify aspects of its guidelines that need updating and revising. As discussed in Chapter 5, however, inconsistencies in guidelines are not necessarily unacceptable.

One particular implementation problem for the Forum and other sponsors of guidelines is ensuring that outdated versions of guidelines are abandoned. To the extent that a set of guidelines have been integrated into the operations of thousands of local organizations and practitioner offices and incorporated into specialized computer software and information systems, this practical element of updating will be a particular challenge. (The analogue in medical practice is the abandonment of obsolete procedures and therapies.) In some cases, only parts of guidelines may need to be withdrawn—for instance, the clinical scope of guidelines may change without much need for modification of other elements.

EVALUATION OF GUIDELINES

The purpose of evaluation is to determine what outcomes—both desired and undesired, anticipated and unanticipated—have occurred as a result of a policy or program (Suchman, 1967). For practice guidelines, the primary outcome variables identified in the legislation are the quality, appropriateness, effectiveness, and cost of care provided to Medicare beneficiaries. However, evaluation that concentrates solely on ultimate outcomes and ignores intervening events may be incapable of distinguishing why a policy succeeded or failed.

This chapter distinguishes two kinds of evaluation—practice evaluation and guidelines evaluation. *Practice evaluation* focuses on health care decisions and interventions using various methods. Some methods, for example, randomized clinical trials, explicitly evaluate the impact of clinical interventions on such health outcomes as mortality, morbidity, and quality of life (Institute of Medicine, 1985; Kanouse and Jacoby, 1988; Kosecoff et al., 1987; Lomas et al., 1989). Other methods, such as those employing medical review criteria and the other practice evaluation tools described in Chapter 2, typically do not assess outcomes but instead compare how actual practices (or proposed practices) match practices set forth in the review criteria or standards. These kinds of assessments assume that there are links between such practices and better health outcomes, although, as much of the quality of care literature makes clear, this is not always a viable assumption.

A second type of evaluation, which is the focus of the following discussion, is better described as a form of *policy and program evaluation*. The question is whether public and private policies and programs in this area have the effects intended; that is, do practice guidelines, as a policy instrument, affect clinical practice and health outcomes? This kind of evaluation can encompass every step in the development and implementation of guidelines and the intermediate outcomes of each of these steps.

Evaluating the impact of guidelines means determining their major intended and unintended effects and, insofar as possible, the causes of these effects (or their absence). A recent survey of practice guidelines activities conducted for the IOM concluded that, among organizations involved with guidelines, implementation and evaluation have received secondary emphasis compared with development and promulgation (Audet and Greenfield, 1989). Relatively few steps were under way or planned to evaluate the impact of guidelines on the cost, quality, and outcomes of care and on patient and practitioner satisfaction. This neglect of evaluation is unfortunate because the effectiveness of guidelines cannot be taken for granted.

Two areas of concern can be raised with respect to the evaluation of practice guidelines. First are narrow issues relating to specific legislative requirements for DHHS. Second are broad questions about how to evaluate the impact of guidelines and build better policies and programs based on that evaluation. This report focuses on the first set of issues.

The necessary planning to meet OBRA 89 requirements should start now. Such planning is particularly important because the legislation's requirements raise several problems, which the committee understands are recognized by department officials and congressional staff. Most simply stated, although the legislation's provisions for evaluation are laudable, the 1993 timetable for evaluating the first three guidelines developed by the Forum is unrealistic. On the one hand, the guidelines probably will not have had time to make a measurable impact. On the other hand, even if the guidelines had had fairly immediate effects, the measurement data to document such effects would generally be unavailable. For example, insurance claims or other data showing changes in the use of procedures or practices may not be accessible in the time frame specified. Likewise, data on patient outcomes will take time to collect.

Rather than ask Congress for a change in the evaluation timetable, the Forum proposes to provide a status report as of January 1, 1993. The committee considers this appropriate so long as DHHS begins serious planning for the evaluation soon and takes steps to put necessary data collection processes in place. As noted earlier, many of the steps needed for evaluation can and should be initially considered and specified as guidelines are developed. Indeed, a hallmark of good evaluation research is that planning for the evaluation begins before the program gets under way. Over the long term, the data development responsibilities of AHCPR can be used to support guidelines evaluation as well as outcomes and effectiveness research.

OBRA 89 requires evaluation of the impact of guidelines on quality, effectiveness, appropriateness, and cost of care. Information on *intermediate outcomes* or *intervening variables* is also important to determine such facts as whether the guidelines have, indeed, been received, read, understood, accepted, and remembered by practitioners and patients (Kaluzny, 1990;

Lomas, 1990). Such information is essential to understanding why a set of guidelines have or have not achieved their desired outcomes and to determining whether to continue, revise, or abandon the guidelines. In general, explanations for policy success or failure need to consider evidence about the following:

- the validity of the policy premises, for example, the assumption of many policymakers that broader development and use of practice guidelines will achieve significant cost savings;
- the quality of the implementation process, for example, the extent to which information was disseminated or incentives were created for the use of the guidelines;
- the existence of countervailing events, for example, court decisions limiting the ability of health care organizations or payers to review the appropriateness of care and then deny either practice privileges or payment for practitioners providing inappropriate care; and
- the nature of supportive or enabling conditions, for example, the breadth of professional interest in the topic covered by the guidelines or a technical breakthrough in access to computer-based information systems.

This chapter has suggested several aspects of the implementation processes for both the government program and the guidelines themselves that warrant assessment. These aspects include (1) the effectiveness of different formats for a given guideline, (2) the impact of different dissemination strategies for different audiences, and (3) the role of alternative means of promoting day-to-day application of the guidelines. Indeed, the entire process of guidelines development will surely need investigation over time. No one approach is, in the short run (if ever), likely to prove definitively superior, although unsatisfactory methods can be identified and the strengths and weaknesses of other methods can be better understood. In addition, evaluation of the cost-effectiveness of different implementation activities could help in making decisions about how to allocate limited government and private resources.

CONCLUSION

The charge to this IOM committee was narrow: to provide timely advice to AHCPR on its initial steps to meet its responsibilities for practice guidelines under OBRA 89. To that end, the committee focused on definitions and attributes for practice guidelines and on certain aspects of guidelines implementation and evaluation. For the latter, the emphasis is on how implementation and evaluation decisions can relate to and reinforce such attributes of guidelines as validity and reliability.

diagnosing, and/or managing selected health conditions" (working definition).

IOM (1990:304): "Appropriateness guidelines describe accepted indications for using particular medical interventions and technologies, ranging from surgical procedures to diagnostic studies."

Joint Commission on Accreditation of Healthcare Organizations (1989a): A guideline gives "indications or contraindications for appropriate patient care."

Physician Payment Review Commission: (1) "Practice guidelines are standardized specifications for care, either for the use of a particular service [e.g., preventive screening] or procedure or for the management of a specific clinical problem" (1988a:13). (2) "[Practice guidelines refer to] formally developed guidelines based on the clinical research literature and the collective judgments of experts" (1988b:223). (3) ". . .[E]ssentially clinical recommendations for patient care. They provide guidance to physicians and others who must make decisions. . ." (1988b:223).

U.S. Preventive Services Task Force (1989:xxxvii): "Recommendations appearing in this report are intended as guidelines, providing clinicians with information on the proven effectiveness of preventive services in published clinical research. Recommendations for or against performing these maneuvers should not be interpreted as standards of care but rather as statements regarding the quality of the supporting scientific evidence."

Mark Chassin (1988): "They [standards of care or practice guidelines] are statements describing specific diagnostic or therapeutic maneuvers that should or should not be performed in certain specific clinical circumstances."

David Eddy (forthcoming): "Pathway guidelines (protocols and algorithms) are intended to direct a practitioner along a preferred management path. Boundary guidelines (limits or criteria) are intended to define the limits of proper practice." In distinguishing different types of practice policies (standards, guidelines, and options), Eddy states: "A practice policy is considered a guideline if the outcomes of the intervention are well enough understood to permit meaningful decisions about its proper use, and if it is preferred (or not preferred) by an appreciable but not unanimous majority of people." (Note in the section below that Eddy requires more stringent agreement for a standard.)

Lucien Leape (1990:43): Practice guidelines are "standardized specifications for care developed by a formal process that incorporates the best scientific evidence of effectiveness with expert opinion."

The committee's basic conclusion is that AHCPR and the Forum must incorporate planning for implementation—formatting, dissemination, application, and updating—and evaluation within their development strategy. For the overall process to be successful, in fact, it may be necessary for the Forum to devote some of its scarce resources now to these more future-oriented needs.

REFERENCES

American College of Physicians. *Clinical Efficacy Assessment Project: Procedural Manual.* Philadelphia: 1986.

Audet, A., and Greenfield, S. A Survey of Current Activities in Practice Guideline Development. Paper prepared for an IOM Meeting on Medical Practice Guidelines: Looking Ahead, Washington, D.C., November 8, 1989.

Avorn, J., and Somerai, S. Improving Drug-Therapy Decisions Through Educational Outreach: A Randomized Controlled Trial of Academically-Based "Detailing." *New England Journal of Medicine* 308:1457–1460, 1983.

Field, M. Health Policy and Medical Practice Guidelines: The Case of Mammography Screening for Women Under 50. Paper prepared for an IOM Meeting on Medical Practice Guidelines: Looking Ahead, Washington, D.C., November 8, 1989.

Greenes, R., and Shortliffe, E. Medical Informatics: An Emerging Academic Discipline and Institutional Priority. *Journal of the American Medical Association* 263:1114–1120, 1990.

Institute of Medicine. Effects of Clinical Evaluation on the Diffusion of Medical Technology. Chapter 4 in *Assessing Medical Technologies.* Washington, D.C.: National Academy Press, 1985.

Institute of Medicine. *Controlling Costs and Changing Patient Care? The Role of Utilization Management,* B. Gray and M. Field, eds. Washington, D.C.: National Academy Press, 1989.

Institute of Medicine. *Medicare: A Strategy for Quality Assurance,* vols. 1 and 2, K. Lohr, ed. Washington, D.C.: National Academy Press, 1990.

Jacoby, I., and Clarke, S. Direct Mailing as a Means of Disseminating NIH Consensus Statements. *Journal of the American Medical Association* 255:1328–1330, 1986.

Kaluzny, A. Dissemination and Impact of Consensus Development Statements. Pp. 69-83 in *Improving Consensus Development for Health Technology Assessment: An International Perspective.* Washington, D.C.: National Academy Press, 1990.

Kanouse, D.E., and Jacoby, I. When Does Information Change Practitioners' Behavior? *International Journal of Technology Assessment in Health Care* 4(1):27–33, 1988.

Kosecoff, J., Kanouse, D., Rogers, W., et al., Effects of National Institutes of Health Consensus Development Program on Physician Practice. *Journal of the American Medical Association* 258:2708–2713, 1987.

Lomas, J. Words Without Action? The Production, Dissemination, and Impact of Consensus Recommendations. In *Annual Review of Public Health,* vol. 12, G. Omenn, ed. Palo Alto, Calif.: forthcoming (draft dated May 1990).

Lomas, J., Anderson, K., Dominick-Pierre, E., et al. Do Practice Guidelines Guide Practice? The Effects of a Consensus Statement on the Practice of Physicians. *New England Journal of Medicine* 321:1306–1311, 1989.

Lundberg, G. Providing Reliable Medical Information to the Public—Caveat Lector. *Journal of the American Medical Association* 262:945-946, 1989.

Moldover, S. NIH Scrambles to Get Out the FAX. *Chevy Chase Gazette,* May 3, 1990.

Physician's Desk Reference, 44th ed. Oradell, N.J.: Edward Barnhart, 1990.

Pressman, J., and Wildavsky, A. *Implementation: How Great Expectations in Washington Are Dashed in Oakland.* Berkeley, Calif.: University of California Press, 1973.

Rubenstein, E., and Federman, D., eds. *Scientific American Medicine*. New York: Scientific American, 1989.

Shortliffe, E. Computer Programs to Support Clinical Decision Making. *Journal of the American Medical Association* 258:61–66, 1987.

Somerai, S.B., and Avorn, J. Principles of Educational Outreach ("Academic Detailing") to Improve Clinical Decision Making. *Journal of the American Medical Association* 263:549–556, 1990.

Steinbrook, R., and Lo, B. Informing Physicians about Promising New Treatments for Severe Illnesses. *Journal of the American Medical Association* 263:2078–2082, 1990.

Suchman, E. *Evaluative Research*. New York: Russell Sage Foundation, 1967.

Vickery, D., and Fries, J. *Take Care of Yourself: The Consumer's Guide to Medical Care*, 3rd ed. Reading, Mass.: Addison-Wesley Publishing Co., 1986.

Williamson, J.W., German, P.S., Weiss, R., et al. Health Science Information Management and Continuing Education of Physicians. *Annals of Internal Medicine* 110:151–160, 1989.

Word of Spinal-Injury Drug Not Getting Out, Group Says. *Washington Post*, April 11, 1990, p. A5.

5

Conclusions and Recommendations

We would consider our effort a success if more people began with the understanding that implementation, under the best of circumstances, is exceedingly difficult. They would, therefore, be pleasantly surprised when a few good things really happened.

Pressman and Wildavsky, *Implementation*

The challenge facing AHCPR and its Forum in the area of practice guidelines is great, calling as it does for swift movement along many paths in territory that is neither well charted methodologically nor well established culturally. The challenge is intensified by the initiative's origins in the acute public and private frustration about ever-increasing health care spending for services of sometimes doubtful value. Expectations for the guidelines initiative are thus very high.

In the context of current activities and hopes for practice guidelines, the basic charge to this committee was narrow: to define terms, to propose attributes of guidelines, and to explore in a preliminary way issues relating to implementation and evaluation. AHCPR needed the committee's recommendations quickly, and the project's short timetable limited its scope and depth. The statements singled out in this chapter as findings, conclusions, and recommendations are those that relate most directly to the committee's charge. Many of the broader issues related to the development, use, and evaluation of guidelines are being examined in a longer IOM project (see Appendix C).

Throughout this report, the committee has sought to emphasize basic principles that should guide the development, use, and evaluation of guidelines. In most case, it has not proposed specific techniques. The choice of techniques—for instance, how to analyze scientific literature or how to provide incentives for the use of guidelines—will depend on practical circumstances too numerous to cover comprehensively in this document.

This chapter summarizes the committee's major findings and conclusions, reviews its recommendations about definitions of terms and attributes of guidelines, and outlines some of the complexities in implementing and evaluating guidelines that need to be kept in mind as guidelines are developed. The chapter closes with some observations about diversity and conflict among guidelines and the challenges facing the new agency.

FINDINGS AND CONCLUSIONS

STATE OF THE ART

The committee arrived at several general observations about the state of the art of practice guidelines development. Most generally, the process of systematic development, implementation, and evaluation of practice guidelines based on rigorous clinical research and soundly generated professional consensus, although progressing, has deficiencies in method, scope, and substance. Conflicts in terminology and technique characterize the field and are notable not just for the confusion they create but also for what they reflect about differences in values, experiences, and interests among different parties. Public and private activities are multiplying, but the means for coordinating these efforts to resolve inconsistencies, fill in gaps, track applications and results, and assess the soundness of particular guidelines are limited. Disproportionately more attention continues to be paid to the development of guidelines than to their implementation or evaluation. Moreover, efforts to develop guidelines are necessarily constrained by inadequacies in the quality and quantity of scientific evidence on the effectiveness of many services.

AHCPR AND THE FORUM

As a consequence of the above factors, AHCPR and the Forum have, at present, a somewhat restricted foundation for their work. In addition, other variables must be taken into account in estimating what the agency is likely to be able to accomplish early in its guidelines effort. Among the more important are the following.

First, although OBRA 89 addresses some concerns about guidelines development, implementation, and evaluation, it appropriately does not describe a precise course of action for the agency. The committee expects that the agency will need time to devise and revise practical, defensible approaches to guidelines development.

Second, given that both the function and the organizational units (particularly the Forum) are new to the Department of Health and Human Services, the legislative timetables for guidelines development and, particularly, evaluation are unrealistically short. Moreover, the Forum has few staff to support the new functions, and this is not likely to change in the near term. In the immediate future, these constraints and complications are facts of life; the agency is acting to meet its deadlines in as timely and meaningful a way as possible. Over the longer run, however, the committee hopes that experience with the practicalities of guidelines development will lead Congress and the agency to moderate the development and evaluation timetables or to expand the resources devoted to the tasks, or both.

Third, within the government, meeting the challenge of developing good practice guidelines cannot be solely the responsibility of the Forum. Other parts of AHCPR, for instance, its Medical Treatment Effectiveness Program (MEDTEP), will surely generate information of immediate importance for practice guidelines. Moreover, the exchange of information among units of government is a two-way process; lacunae in data identified during the guidelines development process should highlight areas that AHCPR can target for research funding. Outside AHCPR, the work of other agencies in the Public Health Service, most notably the National Institutes of Health's randomized controlled trials, will be essential to the long-term utility of guidelines, especially insofar as those trials include broad measures of outcomes important to patients. The agency also needs to maintain close links with HCFA, in part because of certain provisions of OBRA 89 but more importantly because HCFA has data on the Medicare population (and, to a lesser extent, on the Medicaid population) that should be of value in developing, implementing, and evaluating guidelines.

ROLES OF PUBLIC AND PRIVATE SECTORS

Despite the focus of this study on advice to a federal agency, the committee believes that the government's role in arranging for the development of practice guidelines may in the end be fairly modest. The contemporaneous efforts of many different organizations in the private sector may significantly outpace what AHCPR can do. This should be even more true for guidelines implementation, where most initiative must rest with private organizations and individuals. Even when the government does play the principal role in funding and disseminating guidelines on certain topics or clinical conditions, guidelines will be tailored or adjusted by providers, health plans, and others to reflect different patient populations, delivery settings, practitioner skills and attitudes, levels of resources, perceptions of risks, and other factors. The committee expects that the processes of guidelines development, implementation, and evaluation will always need to be pursued by both the public and private sectors.

RECOMMENDATIONS: DEFINITIONS

The committee sought to formulate definitions that, insofar as possible, would be clear, concise, and not tautological; consistent with professional and legislative usage; and practically and symbolically acceptable to important interests. It recommends that the Forum work with the following definitions of the four key terms used in OBRA 89.

PRACTICE GUIDELINES are systematically developed statements to assist practitioner and patient decisions about appropriate health care for specific clinical circumstances.

MEDICAL REVIEW CRITERIA are systematically developed statements that can be used to assess the appropriateness of specific health care decisions, services, and outcomes.

STANDARDS OF QUALITY are authoritative statements of (1) minimum levels of acceptable performance or results, (2) excellent levels of performance or results, *or* (3) the range of acceptable performance or results.

PERFORMANCE MEASURES (Provisional) are methods or instruments to estimate or monitor the extent to which the actions of a health care practitioner or provider conform to practice guidelines, medical review criteria, or standards of quality.

The committee recognizes that these definitions will not resolve all arguments over what these and related terms mean, but it believes these four statements will bring a degree of badly needed clarity and uniformity to the field. Moreover, these definitions can be used by the Forum and, indeed, have already been incorporated into its work.

One underlying premise highlighted by these definitions is that these four terms are not synonymous. Assistance to physicians and patients in making decisions is not the same as tools for evaluating practice. Therefore, although the definitions may evolve, it is important to underscore that these are not equivalent concepts or phrases and should not be used interchangeably.

Not part of the committee's definition of practice guidelines but central to its view of the field is the precept that every guideline should be accompanied by a statement of the strength of the evidence and the expert judgment behind it. The committee has not tried to distinguish types or levels of practice guidelines (for example, Level 1 or Level 2 guidelines), although this may be useful. For now, the committee recommends that every set of guidelines describe the strength of the evidence and consensus so that potential users can make more informed decisions.

RECOMMENDATIONS: ATTRIBUTES OF GOOD GUIDELINES

In proposing attributes of good guidelines, the committee tried to define properties or characteristics that would be compatible with professional use and legislative expectations; clearly defined and justified; and demanding but realistically approachable. Prospective assessments of the guidelines (rather than evaluations of their ultimate impact) should use the attributes as benchmarks for judging the soundness of the guidelines. The focus should be on guidelines as a set rather than as isolated statements.

Creating a practical assessment instrument for AHCPR, based on the attributes below, is one task of a second IOM project on practice guidelines (Appendix C). In this first project, the committee has tried to be sensitive to the challenges involved in moving from abstract concepts to real applications.

The committee recommends that the agency look for the following eight attributes, properties, or characteristics when it assesses the soundness of guidelines. Relatedly, the agency should instruct its contractors and expert panels to adhere to procedures that will produce guidelines in keeping with these attributes.

VALIDITY: Practice guidelines are valid if, when followed, they lead to the health and cost outcomes projected for them, other things being equal. A prospective assessment of validity will consider the projected health outcomes and costs of alternative courses of action, the relationship between the evidence and recommendations, the substance and quality of the scientific and clinical evidence cited, and the means used to evaluate the evidence.

RELIABILITY/REPRODUCIBILITY: Practice guidelines are reliable and reproducible (1) if—given the same evidence and methods for guidelines development—another set of experts would produce essentially the same statements and (2) if—given the same circumstances—the guidelines are interpreted and applied consistently by practitioners or other appropriate parties. A prospective assessment of reliability may consider the results of independent external reviews and pretests of the guidelines.

CLINICAL APPLICABILITY: Practice guidelines should be as inclusive of appropriately defined patient populations as scientific and clinical evidence and expert judgment permit, and they should explicitly state the populations to which statements apply.

CLINICAL FLEXIBILITY: Practice guidelines should identify the specifically known or generally expected exceptions to their recommendations.

CLARITY: Practice guidelines should use unambiguous language, define terms precisely, and use logical, easy-to-follow modes of presentation.

MULTIDISCIPLINARY PROCESS: Practice guidelines should be developed by a process that includes participation by representatives of key affected groups. Participation may include serving on panels that develop guidelines, providing evidence and viewpoints to the panels, and reviewing draft guidelines.

SCHEDULED REVIEW: Practice guidelines should include statements about when they should be reviewed to determine whether revisions are warranted, given new clinical evidence or changing professional consensus.

DOCUMENTATION: The procedures followed in developing guidelines, the participants involved, the evidence used, the assumptions and rationales accepted, and the analytic methods employed should be meticulously documented and described.

The stringency of these attributes, especially taken together, is well recognized. Realistically, neither existing guidelines nor those likely to be developed by the agency in the foreseeable future will "score well" on all eight properties simultaneously; indeed, near-perfect scores may always lie in the realm of aspiration rather than attainment. Nevertheless, the committee wishes to emphasize the importance of working toward practice guidelines that exhibit these characteristics.

RECOMMENDATIONS: IMPLEMENTATION AND EVALUATION

The main work of disseminating and applying guidelines will be in private hands, but as OBRA 89 recognizes, the agency cannot and should not be divorced from implementation. Evaluation will be a major agency concern. The committee's discussions centered on how the processes of implementation and evaluation can reinforce and extend the eight attributes defined above.

The Forum should instruct its expert panels and contractors to keep the challenges and difficulties of implementation and evaluation in mind as they develop guidelines. For instance, the tension between extraordinarily detailed, complex, or sophisticated guidelines and those that can be readily translated into medical review criteria, or into documents understandable by the average patient, has to be recognized and dealt with *during* the development process, not after the fact. Keeping implementation and evaluation in mind means, among other things, the following.

• The credibility of the development process, the participants, and the scientific grounding of guidelines must be clear to intended users.

• A truly multidisciplinary approach to guidelines development will facilitate acceptance and use of guidelines by members of the groups represented and by other, secondary target groups.

• Guidelines should be specific, comprehensive, and flexible enough to be useful in the varied settings and circumstances of everyday medical practice and in the evolving programs to assess the appropriateness of care provided in these settings.

• Guidelines language, logic, and symbols should be easy to follow and unambiguous, so that movement from guidelines statements to educational tools, review criteria, or other instruments is unimpeded.

• The guidelines should specify what information about the clinical problem, the patient's circumstances and preferences, and the delivery setting should be recorded to permit later evaluation of the appropriateness of care (judged against criteria generated from the guidelines).

The Forum can underscore its intent to examine critically and improve its processes and products in at least three ways. First, it should ask its expert panels for feedback on the strengths and weaknesses of the procedures followed. Second, the Forum should pretest the guidelines either on a pilot basis in a real delivery setting or on a set of prototypical cases, or using both methods. Third, it should try to evaluate the effectiveness of intermediate steps (for example, formatting, dissemination) that are necessary if guidelines are to have their intended effects on health practices, outcomes, and costs. Each of these steps can be part of a learning process for the Forum and for other interested parties.

Attention to implementation and evaluation must start during the process of guidelines development; these aspects of the guidelines effort should not be dealt with sequentially. Moreover, many parties must contribute to these efforts, and the processes recommended and adopted over the years will evolve as sponsors and participants become more experienced. Today there is no "one best way" to develop guidelines, although preferable—and unacceptable—approaches can be identified. Finally, the effectiveness of any guidelines in reaching desired cost and quality goals *cannot* be assumed. Useful evaluations of impact will take a real commitment of resources.

This report distinguishes between the implementation of the guidelines program called for in OBRA 89 and the implementation of the guidelines themselves. AHCPR and its Forum have the primary responsibility for the former, but the latter will depend largely on private individuals and organizations and will inevitably be harder to coordinate, monitor, and evaluate. The committee's discussion of implementation in Chapter 4 focuses primarily on issues involved in guidelines implementation. However, the discussion of definitions and attributes in Chapters 2 and 3 speaks to two aspects of program implementation: the committee's work with expert panels and its assessment of the guidelines they produce.

The committee also distinguishes between two kinds of evaluation. One is the evaluation of medical practice. Such evaluations may employ clinical trials and other outcomes-oriented methods, or they may rely on medical review criteria and similar tools that compare actual practice with recommended practice. The other kind of evaluation, considered in Chapter 4, asks about the impact of guidelines on the quality, effectiveness, and cost of care.

The implementation of guidelines is a diffuse, difficult-to-track process that will depend on many factors besides the quality and credibility of the guidelines. These factors include the resources devoted to the different steps in implementation, the incentives for use of the guidelines, and the availability of supportive data systems. Different users will have different objectives, and strategies for meeting particular objectives will vary in their cost-effectiveness and manageability for the parties involved. That is, different objectives may call for different choices among (1) formats (physical layout and logic), (2) dissemination media, and (3) administrative supports for users of guidelines in the form of computer-based information systems, periodic feedback, or standard operating procedures.

The committee also discussed a few broad policy issues related to the use of medical review criteria and other evaluation tools derived from practice guidelines. First, consistent with the recommendations of the 1989 IOM report on private-sector utilization management and observations of the 1990 IOM Medicare quality assurance report, review criteria should be public with respect to their content and their development process. This does not require that subsequently developed software and other administrative tools be public, although public monies should not be used to generate, in the first instance, proprietary products.

Second, when criteria are used to assess quality of care, deny payment for specific services, or take similar steps, an appeals process must be provided. This process must be clearly described to patients and practitioners and be free from unreasonable complexity, delay, or other barriers. The attributes identified by this committee—particularly those of clinical applicability and flexibility combined—may help reduce the need for appeals. The point is that individual, idiosyncratic cases will surely surface, no matter how complex and comprehensive the guidelines are, and these eventualities can best be met with an appeals process.

A third issue relating to implementation of medical review programs is the burden on patients and practitioners. Review organizations should make their review activities as manageable and nonintrusive as possible for all those affected by the guidelines. Such organizations are one contributor to the perceived and real "hassle factor" in medical care, which grows out of burgeoning demands by payers and others for more information and justification for services delivered or proposed. The Forum needs to be sensitive to this issue during the guidelines development phase; it also needs to work with HCFA and other organizations to minimize negative effects from poor translation of otherwise good guidelines into review criteria, from unduly stringent application of such criteria, or both. As noted previously, early involvement of provider groups and respected representatives of review organizations, such as the Medicare PROs, is desirable as one means of enhancing the later manageability of guidelines.

Fourth, review organizations should, insofar as possible, provide constructive information and feedback to physicians and other clinicians. This material, and its mode of presentation, should aim to improve practice rather than punish missteps, a view consistent with the overall strategy proposed by the IOM in its Medicare quality assurance study (1990). Regardless of their form, guidelines will not be successful if they are perceived (correctly or not) as vehicles solely for the external control of an obdurate professional community, and the Forum needs to be sensitive to this point.

With respect to evaluation, the study committee believes that the OBRA 89 timetable is unrealistic. The Secretary of Health and Human Services is due to report on the impact of the first three guidelines by January 1, 1993. It is unlikely that these guidelines would have measurable effects on health care or costs that quickly, and even if they did, it is unlikely that appropriate data on patient outcomes and program costs would be available and analyzed. Instead of a full-fledged evaluation, the agency can more reasonably be expected to provide a report on its evaluation plan, the steps being taken to implement the plan, and any preliminary evidence of impact.

DIVERSITY IN CLINICAL PRACTICES AND GUIDELINES

In its discussions, the committee repeatedly returned to questions of diversity in clinical practice and inconsistency among guidelines. Diversity in clinical practice can be acceptable or unacceptable. It may be reasonable when the scientific evidence to support different courses of care is uncertain. In addition, some degree of diversity may be warranted by differences in individual patient characteristics and preferences and variations in delivery system capacities related to locale, resources, and patient populations. However, even though practice variation based on scientific uncertainty or differences in values may be acceptable, both science and values are open to change. Thus, what is perceived as acceptable diversity in clinical practice may change over time.

Diversity in practice is unacceptable when it stems from poor practitioner skills, poor management of delivery systems, ignorance, or deliberate disregard of well-documented preferable practices. It should not be tolerated when it is a self-serving disguise for bad practices that harm people or waste scarce resources.

Guidelines can clarify what is acceptable and unacceptable variation in clinical practice, but that clarification itself has limits that may lead different groups to different and even inconsistent guidelines. Weak evidence is still weak evidence, although the processes described in Chapter 3 should allow the best use of whatever evidence is available. For example, the more formal methods of analyzing and characterizing evidence can reduce the opportunity for inconsistency arising from poor analysis of evidence. Nonetheless, these methods can still leave room for differences of expert opinion about such issues as whether a flaw in research design "matters" or whether differences in results between two treatment alternatives are "clinically important" or only "statistically significant."

Inconsistency among guidelines can also arise from variations in values and tolerance of risk. People may simply differ in how they perceive different health outcomes and how they judge when benefits enough outweigh harms to make a service worth providing. One way to approach this kind of variation is for guidelines developers to try to establish practitioner and patient attitudes toward different benefits and harms and then identify what is known about the probabilities of those different outcomes. In some cases, the developers of guidelines take the further step of applying their own values, but others considering the guidelines later might look at the same information and perhaps come to different conclusions. Also, for some services and clinical conditions, the developers of guidelines may choose not to recommend one course of action but to lay out alternative courses of treatment that may be appropriate, depending on, for example, the preferences of a patient or the characteristics of a delivery setting or community.

In sum, merely identifying inconsistencies in guidelines says nothing about the legitimacy of those inconsistencies. Some inconsistencies may arise from biased or inept development processes. Some may result from reasonable differences in the interpretation of scientific evidence or in the application of patient, practitioner, or social values. Other inconsistencies may essentially disappear when the rationales for specific recommendations are closely examined. The challenge is to determine which explanation applies. Meticulous documentation of the evidence and rationales for guidelines will make this determination easier.

CONCLUDING COMMENTS

As stated at the outset of this report, this committee believes that AHCPR's practice guidelines effort has real potential to advance the state of the art in this field, strengthen the knowledge base for health care practice, and, hence, improve the appropriateness and effectiveness of health care. The conditions for such success are demanding but not out of reach. In particular, expectations for the agency—and for practice guidelines per se—must be realistic regarding timetables and results. All parties concerned must act in good faith and keep the credibility and accountability of their actions in mind. Strict attention to the scientific rigor of the process is critical as is avoidance of premature closure on a single method of guidelines development. Attention to implementation and evaluation needs to be factored into the development process at an early stage.

Fulfilling the agency's mission and potential will require heroic effort from a small staff, serious commitment from participants in the expert panels, and honest, practical support from the many involved and interested parties. Many conceptual and practical issues remain to be confronted. The undertaking will be strengthened if expectations are sturdily realistic, that is, neither too naively optimistic nor too cynically pessimistic.

Appendix A

The Omnibus Budget Reconciliation Act of 1989

Public Law 101-239, the Omnibus Budget Reconciliation Act of 1989, amended the Public Health Service and Social Security Acts to create the Agency for Health Care Policy and Research. The following is an excerpt from that legislation.

SEC. 6103. ESTABLISHMENT OF AGENCY FOR HEALTH CARE POLICY AND RESEARCH.

(a) IN GENERAL.—The Public Health Service Act (42 U.S.C. 201 et seq.) is amended by inserting after title VIII the following new title:

"TITLE IX—AGENCY FOR HEALTH CARE POLICY AND RESEARCH

"PART A—ESTABLISHMENT AND GENERAL DUTIES

"SEC. 901. ESTABLISHMENT.

42 USC 299.

"(a) IN GENERAL.—There is established within the Service an agency to be known as the Agency for Health Care Policy and Research.

"(b) PURPOSE.—The purpose of the Agency is to enhance the quality, appropriateness, and effectiveness of health care services, and access to such services, through the establishment of a broad base of scientific research and through the promotion of improvements in clinical practice and in the organization, financing, and delivery of health care services.

"(c) APPOINTMENT OF ADMINISTRATOR.—There shall be at the head of the Agency an official to be known as the Administrator for Health Care Policy and Research. The Administrator shall be appointed by the Secretary. The Secretary, acting through the Administrator, shall carry out the authorities and duties established in this title.

"SEC. 902. GENERAL AUTHORITIES AND DUTIES.

42 USC 299a.

"(a) IN GENERAL.—In carrying out section 901(b), the Administrator shall conduct and support research, demonstration projects, evaluations, training, guideline development, and the dissemination of information, on health care services and on systems for the delivery of such services, including activities with respect to—

"(1) the effectiveness, efficiency, and quality of health care services;

"(2) subject to subsection (d), the outcomes of health care services and procedures;

"(3) clinical practice, including primary care and practice-oriented research;

"(4) health care technologies, facilities, and equipment;

"(5) health care costs, productivity, and market forces;

"(6) health promotion and disease prevention;

"(7) health statistics and epidemiology; and

"(8) medical liability.

"(b) REQUIREMENTS WITH RESPECT TO RURAL AREAS AND UNDERSERVED POPULATIONS.—In carrying out subsection (a), the Administrator shall undertake and support research, demonstration projects, and evaluations with respect to—
"(1) the delivery of health care services in rural areas (including frontier areas); and
"(2) the health of low-income groups, minority groups, and the elderly.
"(c) MULTIDISCIPLINARY CENTERS.—The Administrator may provide financial assistance to public or nonprofit private entities for meeting the costs of planning and establishing new centers, and operating existing and new centers, for multidisciplinary health services research, demonstration projects, evaluations, training, policy analysis, and demonstrations respecting the matters referred to in subsection (b).
"(d) RELATION TO CERTAIN AUTHORITIES REGARDING SOCIAL SECURITY.—Activities authorized in this section may include, and shall be appropriately coordinated with, experiments, demonstration projects, and other related activities authorized by the Social Security Act and the Social Security Amendments of 1967. Activities under subsection (a)(2) of this section that affect the programs under titles XVIII and XIX of the Social Security Act shall be carried out consistent with section 1142 of such Act.

42 USC 299a-1.   "SEC. 903. DISSEMINATION.

"(a) IN GENERAL.—The Administrator shall—
"(1) promptly publish, make available, and otherwise disseminate, in a form understandable and on as broad a basis as practicable so as to maximize its use, the results of research, demonstration projects, and evaluations conducted or supported under this title and the guidelines, standards, and review criteria developed under this title;
Public information.
"(2) promptly make available to the public data developed in such research, demonstration projects, and evaluations;
"(3) provide indexing, abstracting, translating, publishing, and other services leading to a more effective and timely dissemination of information on research, demonstration projects, and evaluations with respect to health care to public and private entities and individuals engaged in the improvement of health care delivery and the general public, and undertake programs to develop new or improved methods for making such information available; and
State and local governments.
"(4) as appropriate, provide technical assistance to State and local government and health agencies and conduct liaison activities to such agencies to foster dissemination.
"(b) PROHIBITION AGAINST RESTRICTIONS.—Except as provided in subsection (c), the Administrator may not restrict the publication or dissemination of data from, or the results of, projects conducted or supported under this title.
"(c) LIMITATION ON USE OF CERTAIN INFORMATION.—No information, if an establishment or person supplying the information or described in it is identifiable, obtained in the course of activities undertaken or supported under this title may be used for any purpose other than the purpose for which it was supplied unless such establishment or person has consented (as determined under regulations of the Secretary) to its use for such other purpose. Such information may not be published or released in other form if the

person who supplied the information or who is described in it is identifiable unless such person has consented (as determined under regulations of the Secretary) to its publication or release in other form.

"(d) CERTAIN INTERAGENCY AGREEMENT.—The Administrator and the Director of the National Library of Medicine shall enter into an agreement providing for the implementation of subsection (a)(3).

Contracts.

"SEC. 904. HEALTH CARE TECHNOLOGY AND TECHNOLOGY ASSESSMENT.

42 USC 299a-2.

"(a) IN GENERAL.—In carrying out section 901(b), the Administrator shall promote the development and application of appropriate health care technology assessments—

"(1) by identifying needs in, and establishing priorities for, the assessment of specific health care technologies;

"(2) by developing and evaluating criteria and methodologies for health care technology assessment;

"(3) by conducting and supporting research on the development and diffusion of health care technology;

"(4) by conducting and supporting research on assessment methodologies; and

"(5) by promoting education, training, and technical assistance in the use of health care technology assessment methodologies and results.

"(b) SPECIFIC ASSESSMENTS.—

"(1) IN GENERAL.—In carrying out section 901(b), the Administrator shall conduct and support specific assessments of health care technologies.

"(2) CONSIDERATION OF CERTAIN FACTORS.—In carrying out paragraph (1), the Administrator shall consider the safety, efficacy, and effectiveness, and, as appropriate, the cost-effectiveness, legal, social, and ethical implications, and appropriate uses of such technologies, including consideration of geographic factors.

"(c) INFORMATION CENTER.—

"(1) IN GENERAL.—There shall be established at the National Library of Medicine an information center on health care technologies and health care technology assessment.

Establishment.

"(2) INTERAGENCY AGREEMENT.—The Administrator and the Director of the National Library of Medicine shall enter into an agreement providing for the implementation of paragraph (1).

Contracts.

"(d) RECOMMENDATIONS WITH RESPECT TO HEALTH CARE TECHNOLOGY.—

"(1) IN GENERAL.—The Administrator shall make recommendations to the Secretary with respect to whether specific health care technologies should be reimbursable under federally financed health programs, including recommendations with respect to any conditions and requirements under which any such reimbursements should be made.

"(2) CONSIDERATION OF CERTAIN FACTORS.—In making recommendations respecting health care technologies, the Administrator shall consider the safety, efficacy, and effectiveness, and, as appropriate, the cost-effectiveness and appropriate uses of such technologies.

"(3) CONSULTATIONS.—In carrying out this subsection, the Administrator shall cooperate and consult with the Director of the National Institutes of Health, the Commissioner of Food

103 STAT. 2192   PUBLIC LAW 101-239—DEC. 19, 1989

and Drugs, and the heads of any other interested Federal department or agency.

"PART B—FORUM FOR QUALITY AND EFFECTIVENESS IN HEALTH CARE

42 USC 299b.   "SEC. 911. ESTABLISHMENT OF OFFICE.

"There is established within the Agency an office to be known as the Office of the Forum for Quality and Effectiveness in Health Care. The office shall be headed by a director, who shall be appointed by the Administrator.

42 USC 299b-1.   "SEC. 912. DUTIES.

"(a) ESTABLISHMENT OF FORUM PROGRAM.—The Administrator, acting through the Director, shall establish a program to be known as the Forum for Quality and Effectiveness in Health Care. For the purpose of promoting the quality, appropriateness, and effectiveness of health care, the Director, using the process set forth in section 913, shall arrange for the development and periodic review and updating of—

"(1) clinically relevant guidelines that may be used by physicians, educators, and health care practitioners to assist in determining how diseases, disorders, and other health conditions can most effectively and appropriately be prevented, diagnosed, treated, and managed clinically; and

"(2) standards of quality, performance measures, and medical review criteria through which health care providers and other appropriate entities may assess or review the provision of health care and assure the quality of such care.

"(b) CERTAIN REQUIREMENTS.—Guidelines, standards, performance measures, and review criteria under subsection (a) shall—

"(1) be based on the best available research and professional judgment regarding the effectiveness and appropriateness of health care services and procedures;

"(2) be presented in formats appropriate for use by physicians, health care practitioners, providers, medical educators, and medical review organizations and in formats appropriate for use by consumers of health care; and

"(3) include treatment-specific or condition-specific practice guidelines for clinical treatments and conditions in forms appropriate for use in clinical practice, for use in educational programs, and for use in reviewing quality and appropriateness of medical care.

"(c) AUTHORITY FOR CONTRACTS.—In carrying out this part, the Director may enter into contracts with public or nonprofit private entities.

"(d) DATE CERTAIN FOR INITIAL GUIDELINES AND STANDARDS.—The Administrator, by not later than January 1, 1991, shall assure the development of an initial set of guidelines, standards, performance measures, and review criteria under subsection (a) that includes not less than 3 clinical treatments or conditions described in section 1142(a)(3) of the Social Security Act.

"(e) RELATIONSHIP WITH MEDICARE PROGRAM.—To assure an appropriate reflection of the needs and priorities of the program under title XVIII of the Social Security Act, activities under this part that affect such program shall be conducted consistent with section 1142 of such Act.

PUBLIC LAW 101-239—DEC. 19, 1989   103 STAT. 2193

"SEC. 913. PROCESS FOR DEVELOPMENT OF GUIDELINES AND STAND-   42 USC 299b-2.
ARDS.

"(a) DEVELOPMENT THROUGH CONTRACTS AND PANELS.—The Director shall—
    "(1) enter into contracts with public and nonprofit private
entities for the purpose of developing and periodically reviewing
and updating the guidelines, standards, performance measures,
and review criteria described in section 912(a); and
    "(2) convene panels of appropriately qualified experts (includ-
ing practicing physicians with appropriate expertise) and health
care consumers for the purpose of—
        "(A) developing and periodically reviewing and updating
    the guidelines, standards, performance measures, and
    review criteria described in section 912(a); and
        "(B) reviewing the guidelines, standards, performance
    measures, and review criteria developed under contracts
    under paragraph (1).
"(b) AUTHORITY FOR ADDITIONAL PANELS.—The Director may convene panels of appropriately qualified experts (including practicing
physicians with appropriate expertise) and health care consumers
for the purpose of—
    "(1) developing the standards and criteria described in section
914(b); and
    "(2) providing advice to the Administrator and the Director
with respect to any other activities carried out under this part
or under section 902(a)(2).
"(c) SELECTION OF PANEL MEMBERS.—In selecting individuals to
serve on panels convened under this section, the Director shall
consult with a broad range of interested individuals and organizations, including organizations representing physicians in the general
practice of medicine and organizations representing physicians in
specialties and subspecialties pertinent to the purposes of the panel
involved. The Director shall seek to appoint physicians reflecting a
variety of practice settings.

"SEC. 914. ADDITIONAL REQUIREMENTS.   42 USC 299b-3.

"(a) PROGRAM AGENDA.—
    "(1) IN GENERAL.—The Administrator shall provide for an
agenda for the development of the guidelines, standards,
performance measures, and review criteria described in section
912(a), including—
        "(A) with respect to the guidelines, identifying specific
    diseases, disorders, and other health conditions for which
    the guidelines are to be developed and those that are to be
    given priority in the development of the guidelines; and
        "(B) with respect to the standards, performance meas-
    ures, and review criteria, identifying specific aspects of
    health care for which the standards, performance meas-
    ures, and review criteria are to be developed and those that
    are to be given priority in the development of the stand-
    ards, performance measures, and review criteria.
    "(2) CONSIDERATION OF CERTAIN FACTORS IN ESTABLISHING
PRIORITIES.—
        "(A) Factors considered by the Administrator in
    establishing priorities for purposes of paragraph (1) shall
    include consideration of the extent to which the guidelines,

standards, performance measures, and review criteria involved can be expected—

"(i) to improve methods of prevention, diagnosis, treatment, and clinical management for the benefit of a significant number of individuals;

"(ii) to reduce clinically significant variations among physicians in the particular services and procedures utilized in making diagnoses and providing treatments; and

"(iii) to reduce clinically significant variations in the outcomes of health care services and procedures.

"(B) In providing for the agenda required in paragraph (1), including the priorities, the Administrator shall consult with the Administrator of the Health Care Financing Administration and otherwise act consistent with section 1142(b)(3) of the Social Security Act.

"(b) STANDARDS AND CRITERIA.—

"(1) PROCESS FOR DEVELOPMENT, REVIEW, AND UPDATING.—The Director shall establish standards and criteria to be utilized by the recipients of contracts under section 913, and by the expert panels convened under such section, with respect to the development and periodic review and updating of the guidelines, standards, performance measures, and review criteria described in section 912(a).

"(2) AWARD OF CONTRACTS.—The Director shall establish standards and criteria to be utilized for the purpose of ensuring that contracts entered into for the development or periodic review or updating of the guidelines, standards, performance measures, and review criteria described in section 912(a) will be entered into only with appropriately qualified entities.

"(3) CERTAIN REQUIREMENTS FOR STANDARDS AND CRITERIA.—The Director shall ensure that the standards and criteria established under paragraphs (1) and (2) specify that—

"(A) appropriate consultations with interested individuals and organizations are to be conducted in the development of the guidelines, standards, performance measures, and review criteria described in section 912(a); and

"(B) such development may be accomplished through the adoption, with or without modification, of guidelines, standards, performance measures, and review criteria that—

"(i) meet the requirements of this part; and

"(ii) are developed by entities independently of the program established in this part.

"(4) IMPROVEMENTS OF STANDARDS AND CRITERIA.—The Director shall conduct and support research with respect to improving the standards and criteria developed under this subsection.

"(c) DISSEMINATION.—The Director shall promote and support the dissemination of the guidelines, standards, performance measures, and review criteria described in section 912(a). Such dissemination shall be carried out through organizations representing health care providers, organizations representing health care consumers, peer review organizations, accrediting bodies, and other appropriate entities.

"(d) PILOT TESTING.—The Director may conduct or support pilot testing of the guidelines, standards, performance measures, and review criteria developed under section 912(a). Any such pilot testing may be conducted prior to, or concurrently with, their dissemination under subsection (c).

"(e) EVALUATIONS.—The Director shall conduct and support evaluations of the extent to which the guidelines, standards, performance standards, and review criteria developed under section 912 have had an effect on the clinical practice of medicine.

"(f) RECOMMENDATIONS TO ADMINISTRATOR.—The Director shall make recommendations to the Administrator on activities that should be carried out under section 902(a)(2) and under section 1142 of the Social Security Act, including recommendations of particular research projects that should be carried out with respect to—

"(1) evaluating the outcomes of health care services and procedures;

"(2) developing the standards and criteria required in subsection (b); and

"(3) promoting the utilization of the guidelines, standards, performance standards, and review criteria developed under section 912(a).".

(b) OUTCOMES OF HEALTH CARE SERVICES AND PROCEDURES.—

(1) ESTABLISHMENT OF PROGRAM OF RESEARCH.—Part A of title XI of the Social Security Act (42 U.S.C. 1301 et seq.) is amended by adding at the end the following new section:

"RESEARCH ON OUTCOMES OF HEALTH CARE SERVICES AND PROCEDURES

"SEC. 1142. (a) ESTABLISHMENT OF PROGRAM.—   42 USC
1320b-12.

"(1) IN GENERAL.—The Secretary, acting through the Administrator for Health Care Policy and Research, shall—

"(A) conduct and support research with respect to the outcomes, effectiveness, and appropriateness of health care services and procedures in order to identify the manner in which diseases, disorders, and other health conditions can most effectively and appropriately be prevented, diagnosed, treated, and managed clinically; and

"(B) assure that the needs and priorities of the program under title XVIII are appropriately reflected in the development and periodic review and updating (through the process set forth in section 913 of the Public Health Service Act) of treatment-specific or condition-specific practice guidelines for clinical treatments and conditions in forms appropriate for use in clinical practice, for use in educational programs, and for use in reviewing quality and appropriateness of medical care.

"(2) EVALUATIONS OF ALTERNATIVE SERVICES AND PROCEDURES.—In carrying out paragraph (1), the Secretary shall conduct or support evaluations of the comparative effects, on health and functional capacity, of alternative services and procedures utilized in preventing, diagnosing, treating, and clinically managing diseases, disorders, and other health conditions.

"(3) INITIAL GUIDELINES.—

"(A) In carrying out paragraph (1)(B) of this subsection, and section 912(d) of the Public Health Service Act, the Secretary shall, by not later than January 1, 1991, assure the development of an initial set of the guidelines specified in paragraph (1)(B) that shall include not less than 3 clinical treatments or conditions that—

PUBLIC LAW 101-239—DEC. 19, 1989

"(i)(I) account for a significant portion of expenditures under title XVIII; and

"(II) have a significant variation in the frequency or the type of treatment provided; or

"(ii) otherwise meet the needs and priorities of the program under title XVIII, as set forth under subsection (b)(3).

"(B)(i) The Secretary shall provide for the use of guidelines developed under subparagrah (A) to improve the quality, effectiveness, and appropriateness of care provided under title XVIII. The Secretary shall determine the impact of such use on the quality, appropriateness, effectiveness, and cost of medical care provided under such title and shall report to the Congress on such determination by not later than January 1, 1993.

"(ii) For the purpose of carrying out clause (i), the Secretary shall expend, from the amounts specified in clause (iii), $1,000,000 for fiscal year 1990 and $1,500,000 for each of the fiscal years 1991 and 1992.

"(iii) For each fiscal year, for purposes of expenditures required in clause (ii)—

"(I) 60 percent of an amount equal to the expenditure involved is appropriated from the Federal Hospital Insurance Trust Fund (established under section 1817); and

"(II) 40 percent of an amount equal to the expenditure involved is appropriated from the Federal Supplementary Medical Insurance Trust Fund (established under section 1841).

"(b) PRIORITIES.—

"(1) IN GENERAL.—The Secretary shall establish priorities with respect to the diseases, disorders, and other health conditions for which research and evaluations are to be conducted or supported under subsection (a). In establishing such priorities, the Secretary shall, with respect to a disease, disorder, or other health condition, consider the extent to which—

"(A) improved methods of prevention, diagnosis, treatment, and clinical management can benefit a significant number of individuals;

"(B) there is significant variation among physicians in the particular services and procedures utilized in making diagnoses and providing treatments or there is significant variation in the outcomes of health care services or procedures due to different patterns of diagnosis or treatment;

"(C) the services and procedures utilized for diagnosis and treatment result in relatively substantial expenditures; and

"(D) the data necessary for such evaluations are readily available or can readily be developed.

"(2) PRELIMINARY ASSESSMENTS.—For the purpose of establishing priorities under paragraph (1), the Secretary may, with respect to services and procedures utilized in preventing, diagnosing, treating, and clinically managing diseases, disorders, and other health conditions, conduct or support assessments of the extent to which—

"(A) rates of utilization vary among similar populations for particular diseases, disorders, and other health conditions;

"(B) uncertainties exist on the effect of utilizing a particular service or procedure; or

"(C) inappropriate services and procedures are provided.

"(3) RELATIONSHIP WITH MEDICARE PROGRAM.—In establishing priorities under paragraph (1) for research and evaluation, and under section 914(a) of the Public Health Service Act for the agenda under such section, the Secretary shall assure that such priorities appropriately reflect the needs and priorities of the program under title XVIII, as set forth by the Administrator of the Health Care Financing Administration.

"(c) METHODOLOGIES AND CRITERIA FOR EVALUATIONS.—For the purpose of facilitating research under subsection (a), the Secretary shall—

"(1) conduct and support research with respect to the improvement of methodologies and criteria utilized in conducting research with respect to outcomes of health care services and procedures;

"(2) conduct and support reviews and evaluations of existing research findings with respect to such treatment or conditions;

"(3) conduct and support reviews and evaluations of the existing methodologies that use large data bases in conducting such research and shall develop new research methodologies, including data-based methods of advancing knowledge and methodologies that measure clinical and functional status of patients, with respect to such research;

"(4) provide grants and contracts to research centers, and contracts to other entities, to conduct such research on such treatment or conditions, including research on the appropriate use of prescription drugs;

Grants.
Contracts.

"(5) conduct and support research and demonstrations on the use of claims data and data on clinical and functional status of patients in determining the outcomes, effectiveness, and appropriateness of such treatment; and

"(6) conduct and support supplementation of existing data bases, including the collection of new information, to enhance data bases for research purposes, and the design and development of new data bases that would be used in outcomes and effectiveness research.

"(d) STANDARDS FOR DATA BASES.—In carrying out this section, the Secretary shall develop—

"(1) uniform definitions of data to be collected and used in describing a patient's clinical and functional status;

"(2) common reporting formats and linkages for such data; and

"(3) standards to assure the security, confidentiality, accuracy, and appropriate maintenance of such data.

"(e) DISSEMINATION OF RESEARCH FINDINGS AND GUIDELINES.—

Education.

"(1) IN GENERAL.—The Secretary shall provide for the dissemination of the findings of research and the guidelines described in subsection (a), and for the education of providers and others in the application of such research findings and guidelines.

"(2) COOPERATIVE EDUCATIONAL ACTIVITIES.—In disseminating findings and guidelines under paragraph (1), and in providing for education under such paragraph, the Secretary shall work with professional associations, medical specialty and subspecialty organizations, and other relevant groups to identify and implement effective means to educate physicians, other providers, consumers, and others in using such findings and guidelines, including training for physician managers within provider organizations.

"(f) EVALUATIONS.—The Secretary shall conduct and support evaluations of the activities carried out under this section to determine the extent to which such activities have had an effect on the practices of physicians in providing medical treatment, the delivery of health care, and the outcomes of health care services and procedures.

"(g) RESEARCH WITH RESPECT TO DISSEMINATION.—The Secretary may conduct or support research with respect to improving methods of disseminating information on the effectiveness and appropriateness of health care services and procedures.

"(h) REPORT TO CONGRESS.—Not later than February 1 of each of the years 1991 and 1992, and of each second year thereafter, the Secretary shall report to the Congress on the progress of the activities under this section during the preceding fiscal year (or preceding 2 fiscal years, as appropriate), including the impact of such activities on medical care (particularly medical care for individuals receiving benefits under title XVIII).

"(i) AUTHORIZATION OF APPROPRIATIONS.—

"(1) IN GENERAL.—There are authorized to be appropriated to carry out this section—

"(A) $50,000,000 for fiscal year 1990;
"(B) $75,000,000 for fiscal year 1991;
"(C) $110,000,000 for fiscal year 1992;
"(D) $148,000,000 for fiscal year 1993; and
"(E) $185,000,000 for fiscal year 1994.

"(2) SPECIFICATIONS.—For the purpose of carrying out this section, for each of the fiscal years 1990 through 1992 an amount equal to two-thirds of the amounts authorized to be appropriated under paragraph (1), and for each of the fiscal years 1993 and 1994 an amount equal to 70 percent of such amounts, are to be appropriated in the following proportions from the following trust funds:

"(A) 60 percent from the Federal Hospital Insurance Trust Fund (established under section 1817).

"(B) 40 percent from the Federal Supplementary Medical Insurance Trust Fund (established under section 1841).

"(3) ALLOCATIONS.—

"(A) For each fiscal year, of the amounts transferred or otherwise appropriated to carry out this section, the Secretary shall reserve appropriate amounts for each of the purposes specified in clauses (i) through (iv) of subparagraph (B).

"(B) The purposes referred to in subparagraph (A) are—

"(i) the development of guidelines, standards, performance measures, and review criteria;

"(ii) research and evaluation;

"(iii) data-base standards and development; and

"(iv) education and information dissemination.".

42 USC 1320b-12 note.

(2) REPORT ON LINKAGE OF PUBLIC AND PRIVATE RESEARCH RELATED DATA.—Not later than 1 year after the date of the enactment of this Act, the Secretary of Health and Human Services shall report to the Congress on the feasibility of linking research-related data described in section 1142(d) of the Social Security Act (as added by paragraph (1) of this subsection) with

PUBLIC LAW 101-239—DEC. 19, 1989   103 STAT. 2199

similar data collected or maintained by non-Federal entities and by Federal agencies other than the Department of Health and Human Services (including the Departments of Defense and Veterans Affairs and the Office of Personnel Management).

(3) TECHNICAL AND CONFORMING PROVISIONS.—

(A) Effective for fiscal years beginning after fiscal year 1990, subsection (c) of section 1875 of the Social Security Act (42 U.S.C. 1395ll) is repealed.

(B) Section 1862(a)(1)(E) of the Social Security Act (42 U.S.C. 1395y(a)(1)(E)) is amended by striking "section 1875(c)" and inserting "section 1142".

(c) ADDITIONAL AUTHORITIES AND DUTIES WITH RESPECT TO AGENCY FOR HEALTH CARE POLICY AND RESEARCH.—Title IX of the Public Health Service Act, as added by subsection (a) of this section, is amended by adding at the end the following new part:

"PART C—GENERAL PROVISIONS

"SEC. 921. ADVISORY COUNCIL FOR HEALTH CARE POLICY, RESEARCH,   42 USC 299c.
AND EVALUATION.

"(a) ESTABLISHMENT.—There is established an advisory council to be known as the National Advisory Council for Health Care Policy, Research, and Evaluation.

"(b) DUTIES.—

"(1) IN GENERAL.—The Council shall advise the Secretary and the Administrator with respect to activities to carry out the purpose of the Agency under section 901(b).

"(2) CERTAIN RECOMMENDATIONS.—Activities of the Council under paragraph (1) shall include making recommendations to the Administrator regarding priorities for a national agenda and strategy for—

"(A) the conduct of research, demonstration projects, and evaluations with respect to health care, including clinical practice and primary care;

"(B) the development and application of appropriate health care technology assessments;

"(C) the development and periodic review and updating of guidelines for clinical practice, standards of quality, performance measures, and medical review criteria with respect to health care; and

"(D) the conduct of research on outcomes of health care services and procedures.

"(c) MEMBERSHIP.—

"(1) IN GENERAL.—The Council shall, in accordance with this subsection, be composed of appointed members and ex officio members. All members of the Council shall be voting members, other than officials designated under paragraph (3)(B) as ex officio members of the Council.

"(2) APPOINTED MEMBERS.—The Secretary shall appoint to the Council 17 appropriately qualified representatives of the public who are not officers or employees of the United States. The Secretary shall ensure that the appointed members of the Council, as a group, are representative of professions and entities concerned with, or affected by, activities under this title and under section 1142 of the Social Security Act. Of such members—

"(A) 8 shall be individuals distinguished in the conduct of research, demonstration projects, and evaluations with respect to health care;

"(B) 3 shall be individuals distinguished in the practice of medicine;

"(C) 2 shall be individuals distinguished in the health professions;

"(D) 2 shall be individuals distinguished in the fields of business, law, ethics, economics, and public policy; and

"(E) 2 shall be individuals representing the interests of consumers of health care.

"(3) EX OFFICIO MEMBERS.—The Secretary shall designate as ex officio members of the Council—

"(A) the Director of the National Institutes of Health, the Director of the Centers for Disease Control, the Administrator of the Health Care Financing Administration, the Assistant Secretary of Defense (Health Affairs), the Chief Medical Officer of the Department of Veterans Affairs; and

"(B) such other Federal officials as the Secretary may consider appropriate.

"(d) SUBCOUNCIL ON OUTCOMES AND GUIDELINES.—

"(1) ESTABLISHMENT.—For the purpose of carrying out the duties specified in subparagraphs (C) and (D) of subsection (b)(2), the Secretary shall establish a subcouncil of the Council and shall designate the membership of the subcouncil in accordance with paragraph (2).

"(2) MEMBERSHIP.—The subcouncil established pursuant to paragraph (1) shall consist of—

"(A) 6 individuals from among the individuals appointed to the Council under subparagraphs (A) through (C) of subsection (c)(2);

"(B) 2 individuals from among the individuals appointed to the Council under subparagraphs (D) and (E) of such subsection; and

"(C) each of the officials designated as ex officio members of the Council under subsection (c)(3)(A).

"(e) TERMS.—

"(1) IN GENERAL.—Except as provided in paragraph (2), members of the Council appointed under subsection (c)(2) shall serve for a term of 3 years.

"(2) STAGGERED ROTATION.—Of the members first appointed to the Council under subsection (c)(2), the Secretary shall appoint 6 members to serve for a term of 3 years, 6 members to serve for a term of 2 years, and 5 members to serve for a term of 1 year.

"(3) SERVICE BEYOND TERM.—A member of the Council appointed under subsection (c)(2) may continue to serve after the expiration of the term of the member until a successor is appointed.

"(f) VACANCIES.—If a member of the Council appointed under subsection (c)(2) does not serve the full term applicable under subsection (e), the individual appointed to fill the resulting vacancy shall be appointed for the remainder of the term of the predecessor of the individual.

"(g) CHAIR.—The Administrator shall, from among the members of the Council appointed under subsection (c)(2), designate an individual to serve as the chair of the Council.

"(h) MEETINGS.—The Council shall meet not less than once during each discrete 4-month period and shall otherwise meet at the call of the Administrator or the chair.

"(i) COMPENSATION AND REIMBURSEMENT OF EXPENSES.—

"(1) APPOINTED MEMBERS.—Members of the Council appointed under subsection (c)(2) shall receive compensation for each day (including traveltime) engaged in carrying out the duties of the Council. Such compensation may not be in an amount in excess of the maximum rate of basic pay payable for GS-18 of the General Schedule.

"(2) EX OFFICIO MEMBERS.—Officials designated under subsection (c)(3) as ex officio members of the Council may not receive compensation for service on the Council in addition to the compensation otherwise received for duties carried out as officers of the United States.

"(j) STAFF.—The Administrator shall provide to the Council such staff, information, and other assistance as may be necessary to carry out the duties of the Council.

"(k) DURATION.—Notwithstanding section 14(a) of the Federal Advisory Committee Act, the Council shall continue in existence until otherwise provided by law.

"SEC. 922. PEER REVIEW WITH RESPECT TO GRANTS AND CONTRACTS.   42 USC 299c-1.

"(a) REQUIREMENT OF REVIEW.—

"(1) IN GENERAL.—Appropriate technical and scientific peer review shall be conducted with respect to each application for a grant, cooperative agreement, or contract under this title.

"(2) REPORTS TO ADMINISTRATOR.—Each peer review group to which an application is submitted pursuant to paragraph (1) shall report its finding and recommendations respecting the application to the Administrator in such form and in such manner as the Administrator shall require.

"(b) APPROVAL AS PRECONDITION OF AWARDS.—The Administrator may not approve an application described in subsection (a)(1) unless the application is recommended for approval by a peer review group established under subsection (c).

"(c) ESTABLISHMENT OF PEER REVIEW GROUPS.—

"(1) IN GENERAL.—The Administrator shall establish such technical and scientific peer review groups as may be necessary to carry out this section. Such groups shall be established without regard to the provisions of title 5, United States Code, that govern appointments in the competitive service, and without regard to the provisions of chapter 51, and subchapter III of chapter 53, of such title that relate to classification and pay rates under the General Schedule.

"(2) MEMBERSHIP.—The members of any peer review group established under this section shall be appointed from among individuals who are not officers or employees of the United States and who by virtue of their training or experience are eminently qualified to carry out the duties of such peer review group.

"(3) DURATION.—Notwithstanding section 14(a) of the Federal Advisory Committee Act, peer review groups established under this section shall continue in existence until otherwise provided by law.

"(d) CATEGORIES OF REVIEW.—

"(1) IN GENERAL.—With respect to technical and scientific peer review under this section, such review of applications with respect to research, demonstration projects, or evaluations shall be conducted by different peer review groups than the peer review groups that conduct such review of applications with respect to dissemination activities or the development of research agendas (including conferences, workshops, and meetings).

"(2) AUTHORITY FOR PROCEDURAL ADJUSTMENTS IN CERTAIN CASES.—In the case of applications described in subsection (a)(1) for financial assistance whose direct costs will not exceed $50,000, the Administrator may make appropriate adjustments in the procedures otherwise established by the Administrator for the conduct of peer review under this section. Such adjustments may be made for the purpose of encouraging the entry of individuals into the field of research, for the purpose of encouraging clinical practice-oriented research, and for such other purposes as the Administrator may determine to be appropriate.

"(e) REGULATIONS.—The Secretary shall issue regulations for the conduct of peer review under this section.

42 USC 299c-2.   "SEC. 923. CERTAIN PROVISIONS WITH RESPECT TO DEVELOPMENT, COLLECTION, AND DISSEMINATION OF DATA.

"(a) STANDARDS WITH RESPECT TO UTILITY OF DATA.—

"(1) IN GENERAL.—With respect to data developed or collected by any entity for the purpose described in section 901(b), the Administrator shall, in order to assure the utility, accuracy, and sufficiency of such data for all interested entities, establish guidelines for uniform methods of developing and collecting such data. Such guidelines shall include specifications for the development and collection of data on the outcomes of health care services and procedures.

"(2) RELATIONSHIP WITH MEDICARE PROGRAM.—In any case where guidelines under paragraph (1) may affect the administration of the program under title XVIII of the Social Security Act, the guidelines shall be in the form of recommendations to the Secretary for such program.

"(b) STATISTICS.—The Administrator shall—

"(1) take such action as may be necessary to assure that statistics developed under this title are of high quality, timely, and comprehensive, as well as specific, standardized, and adequately analyzed and indexed; and

"(2) publish, make available, and disseminate such statistics on as wide a basis as is practicable.

42 USC 299c-3.   "SEC. 924. ADDITIONAL PROVISIONS WITH RESPECT TO GRANTS AND CONTRACTS.

"(a) REQUIREMENT OF APPLICATION.—The Administrator may not, with respect to any program under this title authorizing the provision of grants, cooperative agreements, or contracts, provide any such financial assistance unless an application for the assistance is submitted to the Secretary and the application is in such form, is made in such manner, and contains such agreements, assurances, and information as the Administrator determines to be necessary to carry out the program involved.

"(b) PROVISION OF SUPPLIES AND SERVICES IN LIEU OF FUNDS.—

"(1) IN GENERAL.—Upon the request of an entity receiving a grant, cooperative agreement, or contract under this title, the Secretary may, subject to paragraph (2), provide supplies, equipment, and services for the purpose of aiding the entity in carrying out the project involved and, for such purpose, may detail to the entity any officer or employee of the Department of Health and Human Services.

"(2) CORRESPONDING REDUCTION IN FUNDS.—With respect to a request described in paragraph (1), the Secretary shall reduce the amount of the financial assistance involved by an amount equal to the costs of detailing personnel and the fair market value of any supplies, equipment, or services provided by the Administrator. The Secretary shall, for the payment of expenses incurred in complying with such request, expend the amounts withheld.

"(c) APPLICABILITY OF CERTAIN PROVISIONS WITH RESPECT TO CONTRACTS.—Contracts may be entered into under this part without regard to sections 3648 and 3709 of the Revised Statutes (31 U.S.C. 529; 41 U.S.C. 5).

"SEC. 925. CERTAIN ADMINISTRATIVE AUTHORITIES.   42 USC 299c-4.

"(a) DEPUTY ADMINISTRATOR AND OTHER OFFICERS AND EMPLOYEES.—

"(1) DEPUTY ADMINISTRATOR.—The Administrator may appoint a deputy administrator for the Agency.

"(2) OTHER OFFICERS AND EMPLOYEES.—The Administrator may appoint and fix the compensation of such officers and employees as may be necessary to carry out this title. Except as otherwise provided by law, such officers and employees shall be appointed in accordance with the civil service laws and their compensation fixed in accordance with title 5, United States Code.

"(b) FACILITIES.—The Secretary, in carrying out this title—   District of Columbia.

"(1) may acquire, without regard to the Act of March 3, 1877 (40 U.S.C. 34), by lease or otherwise through the Administrator of General Services, buildings or portions of buildings in the District of Columbia or communities located adjacent to the District of Columbia for use for a period not to exceed 10 years; and

"(2) may acquire, construct, improve, repair, operate, and maintain laboratory, research, and other necessary facilities and equipment, and such other real or personal property (including patents) as the Secretary deems necessary.

"(c) PROVISION OF FINANCIAL ASSISTANCE.—The Administrator, in   Grants. carrying out this title, may make grants to, and enter into coopera-   Contracts. tive agreements with, public and nonprofit private entities and individuals, and when appropriate, may enter into contracts with public and private entities and individuals.

"(d) UTILIZATION OF CERTAIN PERSONNEL AND RESOURCES.—

"(1) DEPARTMENT OF HEALTH AND HUMAN SERVICES.—The Administrator, in carrying out this title, may utilize personnel and equipment, facilities, and other physical resources of the Department of Health and Human Services, permit appropriate (as determined by the Secretary) entities and individuals to utilize the physical resources of such Department, and provide technical assistance and advice.

"(2) OTHER AGENCIES.—The Administrator, in carrying out this title, may use, with their consent, the services, equipment, personnel, information, and facilities of other Federal, State, or local public agencies, or of any foreign government, with or without reimbursement of such agencies.

"(e) CONSULTANTS.—The Secretary, in carrying out this title, may secure, from time to time and for such periods as the Administrator deems advisable but in accordance with section 3109 of title 5, United States Code, the assistance and advice of consultants from the United States or abroad.

"(f) EXPERTS.—

"(1) IN GENERAL.—The Secretary may, in carrying out this title, obtain the services of not more than 50 experts or consultants who have appropriate scientific or professional qualifications. Such experts or consultants shall be obtained in accordance with section 3109 of title 5, United States Code, except that the limitation in such section on the duration of service shall not apply.

"(2) TRAVEL EXPENSES.—

"(A) Experts and consultants whose services are obtained under paragraph (1) shall be paid or reimbursed for their expenses associated with traveling to and from their assignment location in accordance with sections 5724, 5724a(a)(1), 5724a(a)(3), and 5726(c) of title 5, United States Code.

"(B) Expenses specified in subparagraph (A) may not be allowed in connection with the assignment of an expert or consultant whose services are obtained under paragraph (1) unless and until the expert agrees in writing to complete the entire period of assignment, or one year, whichever is shorter, unless separated or reassigned for reasons that are beyond the control of the expert or consultant and that are acceptable to the Secretary. If the expert or consultant violates the agreement, the money spent by the United States for the expenses specified in subparagraph (A) is recoverable from the expert or consultant as a debt of the United States. The Secretary may waive in whole or in part a right of recovery under this subparagraph.

"(g) VOLUNTARY AND UNCOMPENSATED SERVICES.—The Administrator, in carrying out this title, may accept voluntary and uncompensated services.

42 USC 299c-5.   **"SEC. 926. FUNDING.**

"(a) AUTHORIZATION OF APPROPRIATIONS.—For the purpose of carrying out this title, there are authorized to be appropriated $35,000,000 for fiscal year 1990, $50,000,000 for fiscal year 1991, and $70,000,000 for fiscal year 1992.

"(b) EVALUATIONS.—In addition to amounts available pursuant to subsection (a) for carrying out this title, there shall be made available for such purpose, from the amounts made available pursuant to section 2611 of this Act (relating to evaluations), an amount equal to 40 percent of the maximum amount authorized in such section 2611 to be made available.

42 USC 299c-6.   **"SEC. 927. DEFINITIONS.**

"For purposes of this title:

PUBLIC LAW 101-239—DEC. 19, 1989   103 STAT. 2205

"(1) The term 'Administrator' means the Administrator for Health Care Policy and Research.

"(2) The term 'Agency' means the Agency for Health Care Policy and Research.

"(3) The term 'Council' means the National Advisory Council on Health Care Policy, Research, and Evaluation.

"(4) The term 'Director' means the Director of the Office of the Forum for Quality and Effectiveness in Health Care."

(d) GENERAL PROVISIONS.—

(1) TERMINATIONS.—

(A) The National Center for Health Services Research and Health Care Technology Assessment is terminated, and part A of title III of the Public Health Service Act (42 U.S.C. 241 et seq.) is amended by striking section 305. 42 USC 242c note.

(B) The council on health care technology established under section 309 of the Public Health Service Act is terminated, and part A of title III of such Act is amended by striking section 309. 42 USC 242c. 42 USC 242n note.

(2) CONTRACT FOR TEMPORARY ASSISTANCE TO SECRETARY WITH RESPECT TO HEALTH CARE TECHNOLOGY ASSESSMENT.— 42 USC 242n. 42 USC 299a-2 note.

(A) The Secretary of Health and Human Services shall request the Institute of Medicine of the National Academy of Sciences to enter into a contract—

(i) to develop and recommend to the Secretary priorities for the assessment of specific health care technologies under section 904 of the Public Health Service Act (as added by subsection (a) of this section); and

(ii) to assist the Administrator for Health Care Policy and Research, and the Director of the National Library of Medicine, in establishing the information center required under subsection (c)(1) of such section 904.

(B) In carrying out section 904(c)(1) of the Public Health Service Act (as added by subsection (a) of this section), the Secretary of Health and Human Services shall, as appropriate, provide for the transfer to the Secretary of any information and materials developed by the council on health care technology under section 309(c)(1)(A) of the Public Health Service Act (as such section was in effect on the day before the effective date of this section).

(C) The Secretary of Health and Human Services shall ensure that the contract under subparagraph (A) specifies that the activities described in clauses (i) and (ii) of such subparagraph shall be completed not later than 1 year after the date on which the Secretary enters into the contract.

(D) For the purpose of carrying out the contract under subparagraph (A), there is authorized to be appropriated $300,000 for fiscal year 1990. Appropriation authorization.

(e) TECHNICAL AND CONFORMING AMENDMENTS.—

(1) SECTION 304.—Section 304 of the Public Health Service Act (42 U.S.C. 242b) is amended—

(A) in subsection (a)—

(i) by striking paragraphs (1) and (2); and

(ii) by striking the paragraph designation in paragraph (3);

(B) in subsection (a) (as amended by subparagraph (A) of this paragraph)—

(i) by striking "the National Center for Health Services Research and Health Care Technology Assessment" and inserting "the Agency for Health Care Policy and Research"; and

(ii) by striking "in sections 305, 306, and 309" and inserting "in section 306 and in title IX";

(C) in subsection (b), in the matter preceding paragraph (1), by striking "subsection (a)," and inserting "subsection (a) and section 306,"; and

(D) in subsection (c)—

(i) in paragraph (1), in the second sentence, by striking "the National Center for Health Services Research and Health Care Technology Assessment" and inserting "the Agency for Health Care Policy and Research"; and

(ii) in paragraph (2), by striking "the National Center for Health Services Research and Health Care Technology Assessment" and inserting "the Agency for Health Care Policy and Research".

(2) SECTION 306.—Section 306 of the Public Health Service Act (42 U.S.C. 242k) is amended—

(A) in subsection (a), by adding at the end the following new sentence: "The Secretary, acting through the Center, shall conduct and support statistical and epidemiological activities for the purpose of improving the effectiveness, efficiency, and quality of health services in the United States.";

(B) in subsection (b), in the matter preceding paragraph (1), by striking "section 304(a)," and inserting "subsection (a),"; and

(C) by adding at the end the following new subsection:

Appropriation authorization.

"(m) For health statistical and epidemiological activities undertaken or supported under this section, there are authorized to be appropriated $55,000,000 for fiscal year 1988 and such sums as may be necessary for each of the fiscal years 1989 and 1990.".

(3) SECTION 307.—Section 307(a) of the Public Health Service Act (42 U.S.C. 242l(a)) is amended by striking "sections 304, 305, 306, and 309" and inserting "section 306 and by title IX".

(4) SECTION 308.—Section 308 of the Public Health Service Act (42 U.S.C. 242m) is amended—

(A) in the section heading, by striking "SECTIONS" and all that follows and inserting the following: "EFFECTIVENESS, EFFICIENCY, AND QUALITY OF HEALTH SERVICES";

(B) in subsection (a)—

(i) in paragraph (1)(A)(i), by striking "sections 304 through 307 and section 309" and inserting "sections 304, 306, and 307 and title IX"; and

(ii) in paragraph (2), by striking "the National Center for Health Services Research and Health Care Technology Assessment" and inserting "the Agency for Health Care Policy and Research";

(C) in subsection (b)—

(i) in paragraph (1), by striking "sections 304, 305, 306, 307, and 309" and inserting "section 304, 306, or 307";

(ii) in subparagraph (A) of paragraph (2)—

(I) in the first sentence, by striking "under section 304 or 305," and inserting "under section 306";

(II) by striking the second sentence; and

(III) by amending the last sentence to read as follows: "The Director of the National Center for Health Statistics shall establish such peer review groups as may be necessary to provide for such an evaluation of each such application.";

(iii) in subparagraph (B) of paragraph (2), by striking "the Director involved," and inserting "the Director of the National Center for Health Statistics,";

(iv) in subparagraph (C) of paragraph (2), by striking "the Directors," and inserting "the Director of the National Center for Health Statistics,"; and

(v) in paragraph (3), in the first sentence—

(I) by striking "section 304, 305, or 306" the first place such term appears and inserting "section 306"; and

(II) by striking "section 304, 305, or 306" the second place such term appears and inserting "any of such sections";

(D) in subsection (d)—

(i) in the matter preceding paragraph (1), by striking "section 304, 305, 306, 307, or 309" and inserting "section 304, 306, or 307";

(ii) in paragraph (1), by striking "in other form, and" and inserting "in other form." and by striking the paragraph designation; and

(iii) by striking paragraph (2);

(E) in subsection (e)—

(i) in paragraph (1), by striking "section 304, 305, 306, 307, or 309" and inserting "section 304, 306, or 307"; and

(ii) in paragraph (2), in the matter preceding subparagraph (A), by striking "section 304, 305, 306, 307, or 309" and inserting "section 304, 306, or 307";

(F) in subsection (f), by striking "section 304, 305, 306, or 309" and inserting "section 304 or 306";

(G) in subsection (g)—

(i) in paragraph (1), by striking the matter after and below subparagraph (C); and

(ii) in paragraph (2), by striking "sections 304, 305, 306, and 309" and inserting "sections 304 and 306";

(H) in subsection (h)(1)—

(i) by striking "section 304, 305, 306, or 309" the first place such term appears and inserting "section 306"; and

(ii) by striking "section 304, 305, 306, or 309" the second place such term appears and inserting "any of such sections"; and

(I) by striking subsection (i).

(5) SECTION 330.—Section 330(e)(3)(G)(i) of the Public Health Service Act (42 U.S.C. 254c(e)(3)(G)(i)) is amended by inserting after "(i)" the following: "except in the case of an entity operated by an Indian tribe or tribal or Indian organization under the Indian Self-Determination Act,".　　Indians.

103 STAT. 2208   PUBLIC LAW 101-239—DEC. 19, 1989

42 USC 11137
note.

State and local
governments.
42 USC 11111.
42 USC 11115.

42 USC 11137
note.

42 USC 299 note.

(6) SECTION 402.—Section 402 of the Public Health Service Amendments of 1987 is amended—

(A) by redesignating subsection (c) as subsection (d) and by inserting after subsection (b) the following new subsection:

"(c) Such Act is amended in section 411(c)(2) by striking subparagraph (B), by striking 'subparagraphs (A) and (B)' in subparagraph (C), and by redesignating subparagraph (C) as subparagraph (B). Such Act is amended in section 415(a) by inserting before the period at the end the following: 'or as preempting or overriding any State law which provides incentives, immunities, or protection for those engaged in a professional review action that is in addition to or greater than that provided by this part'"; and

(B) in subsection (d)(1) (as so redesignated), by striking "subsection (a)" and inserting "subsections (a) and (c)".

(7) SECTION 487.—Section 487(d)(3)(B) of the Public Health Service Act (42 U.S.C. 288(d)(3)(B)) is amended by striking "National Center" and all that follows through "Assessment" and inserting "Agency for Health Care Policy and Research".

(f) TRANSITIONAL AND SAVINGS PROVISIONS.—

(1) TRANSFER OF PERSONNEL, ASSETS, AND LIABILITIES.—Personnel of the Department of Health and Human Services employed on the date of the enactment of this Act in connection with the functions vested in the Administrator for Health Care Policy and Research pursuant to the amendments made by this section, and assets, property, contracts, liabilities, records, unexpended balances of appropriations, authorizations, allocations, and other funds, of such Department arising from or employed, held, used, or available on such date, or to be made available after such date, in connection with such functions shall be transferred to the Administrator for appropriate allocation. Unexpended funds transferred under this paragraph shall be used only for the purposes for which the funds were originally authorized and appropriated.

(2) SAVINGS PROVISIONS.—With respect to functions vested in the Administrator for Health Care Policy and Research pursuant to the amendments made by this section, all orders, rules, regulations, grants, contracts, certificates, licenses, privileges, and other determinations, actions, or official documents, of the Department of Health and Human Services that have been issued, made, granted, or allowed to become effective in the performance of such functions, and that are effective on the date of the enactment of this Act, shall continue in effect according to their terms unless changed pursuant to law.

Appendix B

Examples of Practice Guidelines

Practice guidelines and criteria for reviewing medical care come in a great variety of forms. Although some variations may be merely stylistic, others are linked closely to the intended uses and users of the guidelines. Some developers of guidelines present their products in multiple forms.

To illustrate something of the range of ways in which guidelines are presented, three relatively simple guidelines for breast cancer screening are displayed below in their entirety. In addition, one patient management algorithm is included. The last example is a photostat of the actual algorithm; the other examples have been prepared in layouts and typefaces that closely but not exactly reproduce the originals.

EXAMPLE 1

REPORT OF THE U.S. PREVENTIVE SERVICES TASK FORCE

Screening for Breast Cancer

The first guideline comes from the 1989 report of the U.S. Preventive Services Task Force, a 419-page document intended mainly for primary care providers. The methodology of the 20-member task force was, in many respects, modeled on that of a similar Canadian group first convened in 1976, in which a systematic process and explicit criteria were used to review evidence and develop recommendations. The task force's objective was "to develop comprehensive recommendations addressing preventive services for all age groups" for 60 target conditions.

The report of the group describes its origins, methodology, and participants and includes a set of age-specific charts listing services to be considered during periodic health examinations for patients in seven different age groups. Recommendations for patient education and counseling are also included. After this introductory material, three sections of the report present recommendations related to screening services, counseling, and immunizations/chemoprophylaxis. Within the section on screening services, sets of guidelines related to 47 specific clinical problems are organized as separate chapters. Each chapter follows the approximate format presented in the example below.

SCREENING FOR BREAST CANCER

Recommendation: All women over age 40 should receive an annual clinical breast examination. Mammography every one to two years is recommended for all women beginning at age 50 and concluding at approximately age 75 unless pathology has been detected. It may be prudent to begin mammography at an earlier age for women at high risk for breast cancer (see *Clinical Intervention*). Although the teaching of breast self-examination is not specifically recommended at this time, there is insufficient evidence to recommend any change in current breast self-examination practices.

Burden of Suffering

In the United States in 1989, an estimated 142,000 new cases of breast cancer will occur in women, and 43,000 women will die of this disease.[1] Breast cancer accounts for 28% of all newly diagnosed cancers in women and 18% of female cancer deaths.[1] The age-adjusted mortality rate from breast cancer has been almost unchanged over the past 10 years. Breast cancer is the leading contributor to premature cancer mortality in women.[2] Because women of the "baby boom" generation are now reaching age 40, the number of breast cancer cases and deaths will increase substantially over the next 40 years unless age-specific incidence and mortality rates decline.

Important risk factors for breast cancer include sex, geographic location, and age. Breast cancer is much more common in women than men,[1] and the highest rates of breast cancer exist in North America and northern Europe. In American women, the annual incidence of breast cancer increases rapidly with age, from approximately 20 per 100,000 at age 30 to 180 per 100,000 at age 50.[3] The risk for women with a family history of premenopausally diagnosed breast cancer in a first-degree relative is about two to three times that of the average woman of the same age in the general population.[3-5] Women with previous breast cancer are at increased risk, as are women with a history of benign breast disease.[3,4,6] Other factors with some clinical or statistical association with breast cancer include first pregnancy after age 30, menarche before age 12, menopause after age 50, obesity, high socioeconomic status, and a history of ovarian or endometrial cancer.[3,4,7]

Efficacy of Screening Tests

The three screening tests usually considered for breast cancer are clinical examination of the breast, x-ray mammography, and breast self-examination (BSE). The sensitivity and specificity of clinical examination of the breast varies with the skill and experience of the examiner and with the characteristics of the individual breast being examined. Over the five years of the Breast Cancer Detection Demonstration Project (BCDDP), the estimated sensitivity of clinical examination alone was 45%.[8] Data from studies using manufactured breast models show that mean sensitivity among registered nurses was 65% compared with 55% for untrained women.[8,9] Detection by physicians was 87% for lumps 1.0 cm in diameter, a size comparable to that used in the studies involving nurses and women.[8,10]

Estimates of the sensitivity of mammography depend on a number of factors, including the size of the lesion, the age of the patient, and the extent of follow-up to determine the proportion of "negative" masses that are later found to be malignant (i.e., false negatives). The average sensitivity of the combined clinical examination and mammography in the five years of the BCDDP was 75%. The estimated sensitivity for mammography alone was 71%.[8] A recent report from a multicenter trial estimated the sensitivity of an initial mammographic examination to be about 75%.[11] In a study of 499 women, mammography had an overall sensitivity of 78%, but it was reduced to 70% when only lesions under 1.0 cm in diameter were considered.[12] Sensitivity for all breast cancers in women over 50 was 87%, while sensitivity in women under 51 was 56%. In the 10-year follow-up of a Dutch study, the sensitivity of mammography was 80% for women aged 50 and above and 60% for those under 50.[13]

The specificity of mammography is about 94-99%.[11,13] Even with this excellent specificity, however, false positives can occur frequently if the test is performed routinely in populations with a low prevalence of breast cancer. Thus, most abnormal results of mammograms performed on young women without known risk factors for breast cancer are likely to be false positives. BCDDP data show that only 10% of women with positive (mammography and clinical examination) screening results were found to have cancer,[14] and a recent multicenter trial reported a positive predictive value of only 7% for initial mammographic examinations.[11] There is no study that shows that the sensitivity or specificity of mammography is increased when "baseline" mammograms are available for comparison.

Studies of mammography have shown large variations in observer (radiologist interpreter) performance.[15-17] In a study using 100 xeroradiographic mammograms, including 10 of women with proven cancers, the number of lesions identified as "suspicious for cancer" by 9 radiologists ranged from 10 to 45.[15] In a large breast cancer screening study in Canada, agreement was poor between radiologists at five screening centers and a single reference radiologist.[16]

Because exposure to ionizing radiation can be carcinogenic, widespread testing by mammography has the potential of producing some cases of radiation-induced cancer. However, radiation exposure from mammography has decreased dramatically with the development of dedicated mammography equipment and low-dose techniques.[18,19] Radiation exposure varies with breast size as well as with the specific equipment and technique used.[17-19] Thus, it is important for operators to use low-dose equipment and proper technique to limit unnecessary exposure to ionizing radiation during mammography.

Self-examination of the breast appears to be a less sensitive form of screening than clinical examination, and its specificity remains uncertain. Using reasonable assumptions applied to data from the BCDDP, the estimated overall sensitivity of BSE alone was found to be 26% in women also screened by mammography and physical examination.[8] Estimated BSE sensitivity in the BCDDP varied by age group; it was most sensitive for women 35-39 years of age (41%) and least sensitive for women aged 60-74 (21%).[8] Among participants in a breast cancer registry, BSE was reported to detect 34% of cancers.[8,20]

In a study of women's ability to detect breast lumps, untrained volunteers were able to detect 25% of lumps ranging in size from 0.25 to 3.0 cm in diameter.[8,21] The study showed that the sensitivity of BSE can be improved by training. A 30-minute training session increased the mean lump detection rate to 50%.[21] Although training sessions have increased detection rates, they also increase false-positive rates. False-positive BSE may result in unnecessary physician visits, heightened anxiety levels in women, and increased radiographic and surgical procedures. No study yet reported has directly compared the sensitivity or specificity of self-examination with that of clinical examination and mammography, in part due to the methodologic difficulties with properly designing such a study.

Effectiveness of Early Detection

The results of several large studies have convincingly demonstrated the effectiveness of clinical examination and mammographic screening for breast cancer in women aged 50 and older. The Health Insurance Plan of Greater New York (HIP) in 1963 began a randomized prospective study of clinical examination and mammography in 62,000 women.[22] The follow-up of this group now exceeds 18 years. In women who were over age 50 at the time of entry into the study, mortality from breast cancer in the screened group was more than 50% lower than in the unscreened group at five years. This effect has gradually decreased to about 21% after 18 years.

In the Swedish "two county study," a randomized controlled trial was begun in 1977 using single-view mammograms to screen about 78,000 women every 20 to 36 months.[23] After six years of follow-up, the group of women who were over age 50 at the time of entry showed a significant decrease in breast cancer mortality. A recently reported randomized controlled trial in Malmo, Sweden, found that in 8.8 years of follow-up women aged 55 and older who received periodic mammographic screening had a significant reduction in mortality from breast cancer.[24] In the Netherlands, a screening program of single-view mammography every two years for women over age 35 was introduced in 1975.[25] After seven years, this case-control study showed that mammography significantly reduced the risk of mortality from breast cancer in women 50 and over. A case-control study in Italy also reported a strong inverse relationship between mortality from breast cancer and mammographic screening in women aged 50 and older.[26]

More than 280,000 women in the United States were screened with a combination of clinical examination and mammography during the Breast Cancer Detection Demonstration Project.[27] This demonstration project was not designed as a research study, however, and lacked a control group. Effectiveness was inferred by comparing the outcome among BCDDP participants with that observed in national cancer surveillance programs. These comparisons showed that BCDDP participants had higher survival rates than those of breast cancer cases in national sample groups.[27] The finding of increased five-year survival was confirmed in a recent analysis of the BCDDP data, which also demonstrated that cumulative mortality from breast cancer was 80% of that expected of BCDDP participants without diagnosed breast cancer at the start of the study.[28] Due to the absence of internal controls in the original design of this study, however, it is unclear to what extent these differences were due to selection bias, lead-time bias, and other sources of bias.[29]

Although most authorities agree on the benefits of screening women aged 50 and over for breast cancer, there has been some uncertainty about the effectiveness of mammographic screening in women between the ages of 40 and 49.[29-31] Mammography for women under 50 has not been shown to be effective in reducing breast cancer mortality in the Swedish "two county" trial[23] or the Dutch study,[25] although the follow-up period may not have been of sufficient duration to detect an effect on mortality. The Malmo, Sweden, trial also reported no benefit for women under age 55, but the mean follow-up period was less than 9 years; moreover, 24% of women in the control group are thought to have received mammography outside of the screening program and as many as 26% of women in the intervention program did not attend screening.[24]

Follow-up data from the HIP study suggest that women aged 40-49 who receive periodic mammography and clinical examination may experience a reduction of about 25% in breast cancer mortality, but the investigators and others have not found this difference to be statistically significant.[22,32] Interpretations of statistical significance when analyzing these data are influenced by a number of factors, some of which include the definition of the 40-49 age group (i.e., age at entry into study vs. age at diagnosis), the length of follow-up, and the denominator chosen to calculate mortality (women entering the study vs. cases of breast cancer). The difference in mortality is statistically significant when cases of breast cancer are used as the denominator and age at entry defines the age group.[33] Statistical significance may, however, be less a consideration than clinical significance. Although nearly 28,000 women aged 40-49 entered the HIP trial, after over 18 years there were only 16 fewer breast cancer deaths among screened women (61 deaths) than in the control group (77 deaths), a difference of about 12 in 10,000 women screened.[33,34]

There are few data regarding the optimal frequency of mammography or the age at which to discontinue screening in the asymptomatic elderly. Although an annual interval is widely recommended, a recent analysis of data from the Swedish "two county" study found little evidence that an annual interval conferred greater benefit than screening every two years.[35] Although there are no reliable data on the optimal age to conclude mammographic screening, there are uncertainties regarding the effectiveness of screening beyond age 75 in asymptomatic women with consistently normal results on previous examinations. The incidence of new disease in this population may be relatively low and thus the effectiveness of screening may be limited, but reliable data are lacking.

Although no large study has quantitated the effectiveness of breast cancer screening for women in high-risk groups, it is apparent that these women have a greater probability of developing the disease.[30] If screening can reduce the risk of mortality from breast cancer, there may be a greater effect from screening those in high risk groups, but studies confirming this effect are lacking. Further, established risk factors are present in less than one-quarter of women with breast cancer, so that a screening program restricted to high-risk groups is likely to miss the majority of cases.

Retrospective studies of the effectiveness of BSE have produced mixed results, and BSE has not been studied in a prospective controlled trial with mortality as an outcome.[8] A recent meta-analysis of pooled data from 12 studies found that women who practiced BSE before their illness were less likely to have a tumor of 2.0 cm or more in diameter or to have evidence of extension to lymph nodes.[36] The studies from which these data were obtained, however, suffer from important design limitations and provide little information on clinical outcome (e.g., breast cancer mortality).

Recommendations of Others

The American Cancer Society[37] and the National Cancer Institute[38] recommend monthly BSE and regular clinical examination of the breast for all women; baseline mammography between ages 35 and 40, followed by annual or biennial mammograms from ages 40-49; and annual mammograms beginning at age 50. These recommendations have been supported by other groups such as the American Medical Association,[39] the American College of Obstetricians and Gynecologists,[40] and the American College of Radiology.[41] A joint statement on screening for breast cancer involving many of these organizations is currently being developed under the organization of the American College of Radiology.[42]

In contrast, the Canadian Task Force,[43] American College of Physicians,[44] and other authorities[45,46] support annual clinical breast examinations for all women starting at age 40 but do not recommend beginning yearly mammography until age 50.

The World Health Organization states that there is insufficient evidence that BSE is effective in reducing mortality from breast cancer.[47] Thus, it does not recommend BSE screening programs as public health policy, although it finds equally insufficient evidence to change such programs where they already exist.

Discussion

At this time, there is little doubt that breast cancer screening by clinical examination and mammography has the potential of reducing mortality from breast cancer for women aged 50 and above. Most studies have not shown a clear benefit from mammography in women aged 40-49. Studies that will provide important information on this topic are in progress.[48] In the meantime, it is unclear whether the effects on breast cancer mortality achieved by screening women aged 40-49 are of sufficient magnitude to justify the costs and potential adverse effects from false-positive results that may occur as a result of widespread screening.[34] Until more definitive data become available, it is reasonable to concentrate the large effort and expense associated with mammography on women in the age group for which benefit has been most clearly demonstrated: those aged 50 and above. Annual clinical breast examination is a prudent recommendation for women aged 40-49.

Conclusions about the cost-effectiveness of mammography have not been universally accepted. Charges vary greatly in the United States, but in 1984 they averaged about $80-$100 per procedure.[30] For screening mammography to be widely used, it is likely that this charge would have to be reduced to $50 or less.[49] Even if only $50 were charged per mammogram, surveying all of the women in the United States over 40 years of age would cost more than $2 billion a year.[50] Others have drawn attention to the additional costs of biopsies performed on the basis of false-positive mammography results.[30] There are also concerns about the availability of the large numbers of trained radiologists needed to interpret additional screening examinations.[50,51]

Wide variation is found in the quality and consistency of mammography, as well as in the accuracy of interpretation, radiation exposure, and cost.[15-18,30] Radiation exposure during routine mammography is frequently much higher than the optimal doses or the minimal achievable doses usually quoted.[17-19] All of the above caveats about mammography argue for caution in the recommendation of mammographic screening, as well as for the selection of mammographers who maintain only the highest standards of quality.

The accuracy of BSE as currently practiced appears to be considerably inferior to that of the combination of clinical breast examination and mammography. False-positive BSE, especially among younger women in whom breast cancer is uncommon, can lead to needless anxiety and expense. With the present state of knowledge, it is difficult to make a recommendation about the inclusion or exclusion of teaching BSE during the periodic health examination. The WHO policy, neither recommending new BSE teaching programs nor changing existing ones, appears to be a prudent interim approach pending new data.[47]

Clinical Intervention

Annual clinical breast examination is recommended for all women aged 40 and above. Mammography every one to two years is recommended for all women beginning at age 50 and concluding at approximately age 75 unless pathology is detected. Obtaining "baseline" mammograms before age 50 is not recommended. For the special category of women at high risk because of a family history of premenopausally diagnosed breast cancer in first-degree relatives, it may be prudent to begin regular clinical breast examination and mammography at an earlier age (e.g., age 35). Clinicians should refer patients to mammographers who use low-dose equipment and adhere to high standards of quality control. Although teaching BSE is not specifically recommended at this time, there is insufficient evidence to recommend any change in current BSE practices.

Note: See Appendix A for the U.S. Preventive Services Task Force Table of Ratings for this topic. See also the relevant Task Force background paper: O'Malley MS, Fletcher SW. U.S. Preventive Services Task Force: screening for breast cancer with breast self-examination: a critical review. JAMA 1987; 257:2196-203.

REFERENCES

1. American Cancer Society. Cancer statistics, 1989. CA 1989; 39:3-20.
2. Leads from MMWR. Premature mortality due to breast cancer--United States, 1984. JAMA 1987; 3229-31.
3. McLellan GL. Screening and early diagnosis of breast cancer. J Fam Pract 1988: 26:561-8.
4. Kelsey JL, Hildreth NG, Thompson WD. Epidemiological aspects of breast cancer. Radiol Clin North Am 1983; 21:3-12.
5. Kelsey JL. A review of the epidemiology of human breast cancer. Epidemiol Rev 1979; 1:74-109.
6. Dupont WD, Page DL. Risk factors for breast cancer in women with proliferative breast disease. N Engl J Med 1985; 312:146-51.

7. Seidman H, Stellman SD, Mushinski MH. A different perspective on breast cancer risk factors: some implications of nonattributable risk. CA 1982; 32:301-13.
8. O'Malley MS, Fletcher SW. Screening for breast cancer with breast self examination. JAMA 1987; 257:2197-293.
9. Haughey BP, Marshall JR, Mettlin C, et al. Nurses' ability to detect nodules in silicone breast models. Oncol Nurs Forum 1984; 1:37-42.
10. Fletcher SW, O'Malley MS, Bunce LA. Physicians' abilities to detect lumps in silicone breast models. JAMA 1985; 253:2224-8.
11. Baines CJ, McFarlane DV, Miller AB. Sensitivity and specificity of first screen mammography in 15 NBSS centres. Can Assoc Radiol J 1988; 39:273-6.
12. Eideiken S. Mammography and palpable cancer of the breast. Cancer 1988; 61:263-5.
13. Peeters PH, Verbeck AL, Hendricks JH, et al. The predictive value of positive test results in screening for breast cancer by mammography in the Nijmegen programme. Br J Cancer 1987; 56:667-71.
14. Wright CJ. Breast cancer screening: a different look at the evidence. Surgery 1986; 100:594-8.
15. Boyd NF, Wofson C, Moskowitz M, et al. Observer variation in the interpretation of xeromammograms. JNCI 1982; 68:357-63.
16. Baines CJ, McFarlane DV, Wall C. Audit procedures in the national breast screening study: mammography interpretation. J Can Assoc Radiol 1986; 37:256-60.
17. Gadkin BM, Feig SA, Muir HD. The technical quality of mammography in centers participating in a regional breast cancer awareness program. Radiographics 1988; 8:133-45.
18. Kimme-Smith C, Bassett LW, Gold RH. Evaluation of radiation dose, focal spot, and automatic exposure of newer film-screen mammography units. AJR 1987; 149:913-7.
19. Prado KL, Rakowski JT, Barragan F, et al. Breast radiation dose in film/screen mammography. Health Physics 1988; 55:81-3.
20. Gould-Martin K, Paganini-Hill A, Cassagrande C, et al. Behavioral and biological determinants of surgical stage of breast cancer. Prev Med 1982; 11:441-53.
21. Hall DC, Adams CK, Stein GH, et al. Improved detection of human breast lesions following experimental training. Cancer 1980; 46:408-11.
22. Shapiro S, Venet W, Strax P, et al., eds. Periodic screening for breast cancer. Baltimore, Md.: Johns Hopkins Press, 1988.
23. Tabar L, Fagerberg CJG, Gad A, et al. Reduction in mortality from breast cancer after mass screening with mammography: randomised

trial from the Breast Cancer Screening Working Group of the Swedish National Board of Health and Welfare. Lancet 1985; 1:829-32.

24. Andersson I, Aspegren K, Janzon L, et al. Mammographic screening and mortality from breast cancer: the Malmo Mammographic Screening Trial. Br Med J 1988; 297:943-8.

25. Verbeek ALM, Hendricks JHCL, Hollan PR, et al. Reduction of breast cancer mortality through mass screening with modern mammography: first results of the Nijmegen Project, 1975-1981. Lancet 1984; 1:1222-4.

26. Palli D, Del Turco MR, Buiatti E, et al. A case-control study of the efficacy of a non-randomized breast cancer screening program in Florence (Italy). Int J Cancer 1986; 38:501-4.

27. Seidman H, Gelb SK, Silverberg E, et al. Survival experience in the breast cancer detection demonstration project. CA 1987: 37:258-90.

28. Morrison AS, Brisson J, Khalid N. Breast cancer incidence and mortality in the Breast Cancer Detection Demonstration Project. JNCI 1988; 80:1540-7.

29. Bailar JC. Mammography before age 50 years? An editorial. JAMA 1988; 259:1548-9.

30. Eddy DM, Hasselblad V, McGivney W, et al. The value of mammography screening in women under age 50 years. JAMA 1988; 259:1512-9.

31. Dodd GS, Taplin S. Is screening mammography routinely indicated for women between 40 and 50 years of age? J Fam Pract 1988; 27:313-20.

32. Day NE, Baines CJ, Chamberlain J, et al. UICC project on screening for cancer: report of the workshop on screening for breast cancer. Int J Cancer 1986; 38:303-8.

33. Chu KC, Smart CR, Tarone RE. Analysis of breast cancer mortality and stage distribution by age for the Health Insurance Plan clinical trial. JNCI 1988; 80:1125-32.

34. Eddy DM. Breast cancer screening (letter). JNCI 1989; 81:234-5.

35. Tabar L, Faberberg G, Day NE, et al. What is the optimum interval between mammographic screening examinations? An analysis based on the latest results of the Swedish two-county breast cancer screening trial. Int J Cancer 1987; 55:547-51.

36. Hill D, White V, Jolley D, et al. Self examination of the breast: is it beneficial? Meta-analysis of studies investigating breast self examination and extent of disease in patients with breast cancer. Br Med J 2988; 297:271-5.

37. American Cancer Society. Summary of current guidelines for the cancer-related checkup: recommendations. New York: American Cancer Society, 1988.

38. National Cancer Institute. Working guidelines for early detection: rationale and supporting evidence to decrease mortality. Bethesda, Md.: National Cancer Institute, 1987.
39. American Medical Association. Mammography screening in asymptomatic women 40 years and older (Resolution 93, I-87). Report of the Council on Scientific Affairs, Report F (A-88). Chicago, Ill.: American Medical Association, 1988.
40. American College of Obstetricians and Gynecologists. Standards for obstetric-gynecologic services, 6th ed. Washington, D.C.: American College of Obstetricians and Gynecologists, 1985.
41. American College of Radiology. Policy statement: guidelines for mammography. Reston, Va.: American College of Radiology, 1982.
42. Dodd GD, American College of Radiology. Personal communication, February 1989.
43. Canadian Task Force on the Periodic Health Examination. The periodic health examination: 2. 1985 update. Can Med Assoc J 1986; 134:724-9.
44. American College of Physicians. The use of diagnostic tests for screening and evaluating breast lesions. Ann Intern Med 1985; 103:147-51.
45. Baines CJ. Breast-cancer screening: current evidence on mammography and implications for practice. Can Fam Physician 1987; 33:915-22.
46. Frame PS. A critical review of adult health maintenance. Part 3. Prevention of cancer. J Fam Pract 1986; 22:511-20.
47. World Health Organization. Self-examination in the early detection of breast cancer. Bull WHO 1984; 62:861-9.
48. Miller AB. Screening for breast cancer. Breast Cancer Res Treat 1983; 3:143-56.
49. Sickles EA, Weber WN, Galvin HB, et al. Mammographic screening: how to operate successfully at low cost. Radiology 1986; 160:95-7.
50. Dodd GS. The history and present status of radiographic screening for breast carcinoma. Cancer [Suppl 7] 1987; 1:671-4.
51. Bassett LW, Diamond JJ, Gold RH, et al. Survey of mammography practices. AJR 1987; 149:1149.

EXAMPLE 2

AMERICAN COLLEGE OF PHYSICIANS

Screening for Breast Cancer

The guideline on screening for breast cancer, approved April 1989, is a product of the Clinical Efficacy Assessment Project (CEAP), an internally funded practice evaluation activity of the American College of Physicians. This project has evaluated laboratory tests, other technologies, and medical procedures and practices and made recommendations in the form of statements or guidelines. A procedures manual for the project, published in 1986, describes 10 elements involved in the CEAP's guidelines development process: identification of technologies as candidates for evaluation, criteria for selecting technologies to be evaluated, selection of consultants, evaluation process, definition of terms, development of statement, review of statement, ratification process, dissemination of statement, and reconsideration of previously approved statements. The primary audience is the College's 68,000 members, who are specialists in internal medicine.

The ACP publishes guidelines in freestanding form as shown below and also has published some sets of related guidelines in manual form. Eventually, the College will publish a comprehensive volume of guidelines, background papers, and other relevant materials. As the guideline shown below illustrates, the freestanding guidelines do not describe the CEAP process, nor do they cite the extensive scientific background papers that are a key element in the evaluation process. For the breast cancer screening guideline, the background paper was prepared by David M. Eddy and published (as are many such papers) in 1989 in the *Annals of Internal Medicine*.

Independence Mall West, Sixth Street at Race, Philadelphia, PA 19106-1572, Tel 215-351-2400

American College of Physicians   *Clinical*
                                                            Efficacy
                        SCREENING FOR BREAST CANCER   *Assessment*
                                                            Project
Disease:

The majority of breast cancers are infiltrating ductal carcinomas; the remainder are of various pathologic types. Although prognosis varies slightly with pathologic type, the principles of screening and management do not differ.

Risk factors for breast cancer include socioeconomic factors, personal or family history, marital status, multiparity, age at first pregnancy, age at menarche and menopause, history of benign breast conditions, and diet.

Screening test(s):

Two main tests are used for breast cancer screening: breast physical examination and mammography.

A breast physical examination performed by a trained practitioner entails visual inspection and manual palpation of the breast.

Two types of mammography are used for breast cancer screening: plain-film and xeromammography. Xeromammography is effective in identifying microcalcifications associated with early breast cancers; plain-film mammography is more effective at detecting poorly defined lesions.

Recommendations:

1. Screening with breast physical examination is recommended annually for asymptomatic women age 40 and older.

2. Screening with breast physical examination and mammography is recommended annually for asymptomatic women age 50 and older.

3. Screening with breast physical examination and mammography is recommended annually for women at any age who have a personal history of breast cancer.

4. Screening with breast physical examination and mammography is recommended annually for women age 40 or older who have a family history of breast cancer or who are otherwise at increased risk.

Rationale:

There is substantial direct evidence that breast cancer screening with breast physical examination and mammography reduces mortality from breast cancer in women over the age of 50. The evidence of effectiveness of mammography for women under age 50 is conflicting; however, the natural history of breast cancer in women under age 50 is such that annual screening with mammography in women who are at increased risk is strongly recommended. All women should be counselled regarding the benefits, risks and costs so they might choose the screening strategy that suits their personal history and preferences.

The risks associated with breast cancer screening are primarily due to false-positive results which can lead to further diagnostic tests, including breast biopsy. Although radiation might increase the risk of a new cancer, the carcinogenic effect of the radiation from mammography is extremely small.

Board of Regents
Approved 4/10/89

EXAMPLE 3

GROUP HEALTH COOPERATIVE OF PUGET SOUND, INC.

Screening for Breast Cancer

The third guideline is taken from the *Preventive Care Manual* of the Group Health Cooperative of Puget Sound (GHCPS), a manual intended "to help physicians and nurses. . .provide comprehensive preventive health care to [GHCPS] enrollees." The introduction to the manual describes how the Group Health Medical Staff Committee on Prevention evaluates screening tests and preventive interventions before they are recommended by the committee for general use in GHCPS. The manual was first compiled in 1987 as a draft document and is being revised on an ongoing basis.

The major part of the manual consists of summaries of the committee's recommendations. The breast cancer screening statement presented below is one such summary. The manual is organized into separate sections on adult screening tests and interventions, pediatric screening tests and interventions, and immunizations. It also includes other information such as a bibliography and removable summary charts that allow quick reference for such information as well-adult screening schedules and general immunization guidelines.

GHC PREVENTIVE CARE MANUAL

Subject:	Adult Screen		Committee on Prevention
	BREAST CANCER	July, 1990 - Update	Reviewed - 1983, 1988

PURPOSE: Early detection of breast cancer reduces mortality in women over 50 and reduces the morbidity of treatment.

WHO: **All women ages 40 and above,** depending on risk factors, with increasing frequency and using additional procedures as one gets older.

PROCEDURE: BREAST SELF EXAM (BSE): Patients are taught to examine their own breasts monthly. The procedure should be reviewed with the patient at the time of professional breast exams.

PROFESSIONAL BREAST EXAM (PE): A thorough exam by M.D. or other trained practitioner. Goal is to detect any abnormalities that warrant further investigation.

MAMMOGRAPHY: An X-Ray study of the breast capable of detecting up to 80 - 85% of cancers.

WHEN: BSE - Monthly - All women should be instructed in BSE, usually at the time of PE (see below) and encouraged to perform the examination monthly.

PE - Annually - During the course of a clinic visit, and as part of a comprehensive evaluation at the Breast Cancer Screening Program Center (BCSPC).

Mammography: Women age less than 40 may be referred for mammography if deemed clinically advisable by their physician. Invitations to women age 40 or more to attend the BCSPC for a comprehensive breast evaluation, including mammography will be scheduled according to the following risk protocol.

RISK PROTOCOL

Mammography Interval	**Women Age 40-49**	**Women Age 50 & Over**
One Year	Previous abnormal biopsy (atypia) OR two or more 1st degree relatives with breast cancer (mother, daughter, sister).	As for women 40-49
Two Years	One 1st degree relative with breast cancer.	One 1st degree relative with breast cancer OR at least two minor risk factors.
Three Years	At least one minor risk factor.	All other women.
Not Recommended	No risk factors.	——

MINOR RISK FACTORS

- Aunt, and/or grandmother with breast cancer
- Menarche age 10 or younger and/or menopause age 55 or older
- No births OR first birth age 30 or older
- Previous negative breast biopsy

Subject:	Adult Screen		Committee on Prevention
	BREAST CANCER	July, 1990 - Update	Reviewed - 1983, 1988

FOLLOW UP: Women with abnormalities detected through the GHC breast cancer screening program will be followed through the program. The primary care physician will be kept informed. Other patients with abnormal findings on BSE or PE should be managed by their primary MD including referral for surgical evaluation when indicated.

COMMENTS: Under the provisions of the GHC risk protocol, 83 percent of all women and 100 percent of all women above age 49, will have mammography at some interval. The percent of women in each screening interval group and their estimated relative risks of developing breast cancer are shown in the table below. The risk algorithm and cancer outcomes from the program are being scientifically evaluated.

At present it remains the physicians' prerogative to order a screening mammogram outside the Breast Cancer Screening Program. Women with a history of breast cancer should get annual mammography through their primary care physician.

Mammography Interval	Percent of Women	Estimated Relative Risk
One Year	3%	4-14
Two Years	17%	1.9-3.5
Three Years	63%	1.2-1.9
Not Recommended	17%	1.0

References:

1. Carter AP, Thompson RS, Bourdeau RV: A clinically effective Breast Cancer Screening Program can be cost-effective too. Prev Med, 1987;16:29-34.
2. Taplin SH, Anderman C: Risk-based breast cancer screening in an HMO: The first year's experience. Group Health Institute Proceedings, June 1987.
3. Thompson RS, Taplin SH, Carter AP, Schnitzer F, Anderman C, Anderson E, White E, Wagner EH: A risk-based breast cancer screening program. HMO Practice 1988;2:177-191.
4. Taplin SH, Anderman C, Grothaus L: Breast cancer risk and participation in mammographic screening. Am J Pub Health, 1989;79:1494-1498.
5. Thompson RS, Taplin S, Carter AP, Schnitzer F: Cost effectiveness in program delivery. Cancer, Dec.15,1989;Supplement:2682-2689.
6. Taplin S, Thompson RS, Schnitzer F, Anderman CA, Immanuel V: Revisions in the Risk-Based Breast Cancer Screening Program at Group Health Cooperative, (Cancer, in press for August, 1990).

EXAMPLE 4

HARVARD COMMUNITY HEALTH PLAN

Dysuria Algorithm

The Harvard Community Health Plan (HCHP) is a multisite, group-model HMO. Over the past several years, HCHP has developed an extensive series of computer-accessible algorithms for ambulatory care management. Each algorithm is developed by a task force of clinicians based on a thorough review of the scientific literature. The task forces operate under the guidance of a research faculty and staff who are experienced in algorithm development.

Each algorithm is followed by explanatory notes regarding options, patients at special risk, and recommended medications and dosages. Some algorithms are several pages long. The HCHP dysuria algorithm is reproduced below.

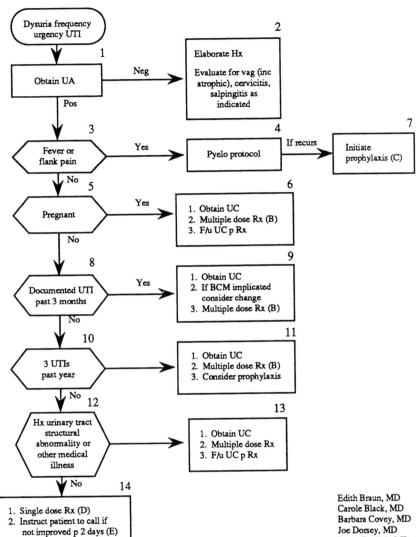

Dysuria frequency urgency UTI

1. Obtain UA — Pos / Neg

2. Elaborate Hx — Evaluate for vag (inc atrophic), cervicitis, salpingitis as indicated

3. Fever or flank pain — Yes / No

4. Pyelo protocol — If recurs

7. Initiate prophylaxis (C)

5. Pregnant — Yes / No

6. 1. Obtain UC 2. Multiple dose Rx (B) 3. F/u UC p Rx

8. Documented UTI past 3 months — Yes / No

9. 1. Obtain UC 2. If BCM implicated consider change 3. Multiple dose Rx (B)

10. 3 UTIs past year — No

11. 1. Obtain UC 2. Multiple dose Rx (B) 3. Consider prophylaxis

12. Hx urinary tract structural abnormality or other medical illness — No

13. 1. Obtain UC 2. Multiple dose Rx 3. F/u UC p Rx

14. 1. Single dose Rx (D) 2. Instruct patient to call if not improved p 2 days (E)

HCHP clinical guidelines are designed to assist clinicians by providing an analytical framework for the evaluation and treatment of the more common problems of HCHP patients. They are not intended either to replace a clinician's clinical judgement or to establish a protocol for all patients with a particular condition. It is understood that some patients will not fit the clinical conditions contemplated by a guideline and that a guideline will rarely establish the only appropriate approach to a problem.

Edith Braun, MD
Carole Black, MD
Barbara Covey, MD
Joe Dorsey, MD
Larry Gottlieb, MD
Talia Herman, MD
Beth Ingram, PA
Carl Isihara, MD
Mon Kim, MD
Tom Lawrence, MD
Carmi Margolis, MD
Marvin Packer, MD
Barbara Stewart, MD

ACUTE DYSURIA IN THE ADULT FEMALE

A. A primary goal of this algorithm is to separate women with acute uncompli-
cated UTI that can be treated with single dose antibiotic therapy from women
with complicated UTI that will require further evaluation or longer duration of
therapy. Therefore, women who have symptoms longer than 2 or 3 days,
women who have fever or flank pain, pregnant women and women with frequent recurrences or other underlying medical problems need to be eliminated
from this algorithm. Initial steps in their management are suggested at branch
points of this algorithm, but other algorithms will be necessary to more fully
address the management of these groups of patients.

Stamm, W., Causes of the Acute Urethral Syndrome in Women, NEJM 1980; 303;
409-415.

B. Choices for multiple dose Rx include 7-10 day course of:

1. Trimethoprim sulfa DS BID (contraindicated in pregnancy, known G6PD
deficiency or allergic Hx).
2. Amoxicillin 250 mg po tid (1st choice in pregnancy).
3. Nitrofurantoin 50 mg QID (alternative for patient with multiple allergies
or pregnant patient with Hx Pen allergy).

C. Prophylaxis is usually continued for 6 months.

Options for prophylaxis include:

1. Trimethoprim sulfa 1/2 regular strength tab, QHS.
2. Nitrofurantoin 50 mg QHS (in pregnant patient or patient with Hx T/X
allergy or known G6PD deficiency).

Ronald, A. and Harding, G., Urinary Infection Prophylaxis in Women, Annals Int.
Med. 1981; 94(2) 268-269.

D. Options for single dose Rx include:

1. Trimethoprim sulfa DS 2 tabs x 1.
2. Amoxicillin 3 gm po x 1.

Kamaroff, A., Acute Dysuria in Women, NEJM 1984; 310; 368-375.

E. Patients who have failed single dose Rx should be considered to have upper
tract infection and treated per pyelo protocol.

SOURCE: Harvard Community Health Plan, used with permission (abbreviations and other details as in original).

Appendix C

Next Steps for the Institute of Medicine

In May 1990, a new committee of the Institute of Medicine (IOM) began an 18-month study of the development, implementation, evaluation, and revision of clinical practice guidelines. The report will cover both public- and private-sector activities.

Many of the issues raised by the IOM Committee to Advise the Public Health Service on Clinical Practice Guidelines will be examined in depth during this second project. In preparing its report and recommendations, the new committee will

- describe existing initiatives to develop, implement, and evaluate practice guidelines;
- identify the strengths and limitations of these efforts in light of the objectives and concerns of specific interest groups and society in general;
- describe different models of public and private action that might serve as prototypes for better structuring activities related to guidelines;
- analyze and assess the strengths, weaknesses, uncertainties, and trade-offs of different models in responding to identified problems and objectives; and
- propose a framework for better structuring the development, implementation, evaluation, and revision of practice guidelines.

In addition, the committee will propose a practical methodology for AHCPR and others to employ in assessing guidelines before recommending or using them. This methodology will focus on the process by which the guidelines were developed, their scientific basis, their relevance to clinical practice, their clarity, and other characteristics. Such initial assessments will not substitute for later evaluations by government and others of the impact of guidelines.

The committee's recommendations will identify legislative, management, and other steps necessary to implement the recommendations. That is, the design plan will propose, insofar as possible, both what to do and how to do it. An active program of disseminating the committee's findings and recommendations is planned. This next project on practice guidelines is supported by grants from the John A. Hartford Foundation, Inc., and the Public Health Service. The committee is chaired by Jerome H. Grossman, and the study director is Marilyn J. Field. The report should be released in the fall of 1991.

Appendix D

Biographies of Committee Members

JEROME H. GROSSMAN, M.D., is the chairman and chief executive officer of the New England Medical Center, Inc. He is also chairman of the Institute for the Advancement of Health and Medical Care and professor of medicine at Tufts University School of Medicine. He serves as trustee/director of several corporations and institutions, including the Federal Reserve Bank, the Boston Private Industry Council, Tufts Associated Health Plan, Wellesley College, and Arthur D. Little, Inc. Dr. Grossman joined the staff of Massachusetts General Hospital in 1966, where he served in a variety of positions. He came to the New England Medical Center in 1979. Dr. Grossman was one of the original staff of the Harvard Community Health Plan, where he developed the world's first automated medical record system, known today as COSTAR. From 1982 to 1987 Dr. Grossman served as program director of the Commonwealth Fund Task Force on Academic Health Centers. He is a member of the Institute of Medicine.

HUGH P. H. BOWER, M.D., was trained in England and has practiced medicine in four countries. For the last 25 years he has been a family physician in rural New Hampshire and Vermont. He is on the board of the American Academy of Family Physicians (AAFP) and three years ago helped to start their Task Force for Clinical Policies. He is also on the Task Force for Clinical Policies for the Council of Medical Specialties Society. He has been chairman of the Committee on Aging of the AAFP for the last two years.

151

ROBERT H. BROOK, M.D., Sc.D., F.A.C.P., is deputy director of the Health Program and a corporate fellow at the RAND Corporation and chief of the Division of Geriatrics and Professor of Medicine and of Public Health at the UCLA Center for the Health Sciences. At RAND he was the leader of the Health and Quality Group on the $80 million RAND Health Insurance Experiment and was the co-principal investigator on the Health Services Utilization Study, which both developed a method to assess appropriateness of care and then applied it to carotid endarterectomy, coronary angiography, and endoscopy. He was the co-principal investigator on the only national study that has investigated, at a clinical level, the impact of DRGs on quality and outcome of acute hospital care. At UCLA he is the director of the Robert Wood Johnson Clinical Scholars Program. Dr. Brook's special research interests include quality assessment and assurance; the development and use of health status measurements in health policy; the efficiency and effectiveness of medical care; and the variation in use of selected services by geographic area. He is a member of the Institute of Medicine, the American Society for Clinical Investigation, and the American Association of Physicians. He recently was awarded the Baxter Foundation Prize for excellence in health services research and the Rosenthal Foundation Award of the American College of Physicians for contributions to improving the health of the nation. He is the author of more than 250 articles on quality of care.

ARTHUR J. DONOVAN, M.D., is professor and chairman of the department of surgery at the University of Southern California in Los Angeles. A graduate of Tufts University School of Medicine, he received his education in surgery at Yale University. Prior to his present appointment, he served on the faculty in surgery at Tufts University School of Medicine, the University of Southern California, and the University of South Alabama in Mobile. At that institution, he was also acting dean and vice president for health affairs. Dr. Donovan has served on the American Board of Surgery, the American Board of Family Practice, and the Residency Review Committee for Surgery. He was chairman of the American Board of Surgery from 1986 to 1988. Dr. Donovan was chairman of the board of governors of the American College of Surgeons from 1987 to 1989. He represented the American Surgical Association on the Council of Academic Societies of the American Association of Medical Colleges from 1979 to 1984. He served from 1982 to 1987 on the Task Force on Academic Health Centers of the Commonwealth Fund.

DAVID M. EDDY, M.D., Ph.D., is the J. Alexander McMahon Professor of Health Policy and Management at Duke University. He received his M.D. degree from the University of Virginia and a Ph.D. in engineering-economic systems (applied mathematics) at Stanford. After serving on the faculty at Stanford as professor of engineering and medicine, in 1981 he went to Duke University to set up the Center for Health Policy Research and Education. Dr. Eddy's research has focused on developing and applying methods for evaluating health practices and designing practice policies. He has developed policies for a number of organizations, including the American Cancer Society, the National Cancer Institute, the World Health Organization, the Congressional Office of Technology Assessment, the Blue Cross and Blue Shield Association (BCBSA), and the American Medical Association. His mathematical model of cancer screening was awarded the Lanchester Prize, the top award in the field of operations research. He recently completed a manual on methods for designing practice policies, a book that describes a new set of statistical methods for synthesizing experimental and nonexperimental evidence to estimate the effect of medical interventions on health outcomes. Dr. Eddy is the methodological consultant to the BCBSA's medical advisory panel, which recommends coverage policies to the BCBSA plans, and is scientific director of the Association's new program to promote quality of care. He serves on the Board of Mathematics of the National Academy of Sciences and is a member of the National Academy of Sciences and the Institute of Medicine.

RICHARD D. FLOYD, M.D., is a general, vascular, and thoracic surgeon at the Lexington Clinic in Lexington, Kentucky. He was chairman of the Lexington Clinic Board of Directors for 12 years. He is a clinical associate professor of surgery at the University of Kentucky. He served as a director of the American Board of Surgery and governor of the American College of Surgeons and has been a member of the board of trustees at Transylvania University for 19 years. He is a member of many surgical societies including the American College of Surgeons and the Southern Surgical Association.

ALICE G. GOSFIELD, J.D., is an attorney from Philadelphia who has worked on legal aspects of utilization management, quality assurance, and peer review issues since 1973. She has been a public member of a statewide Professional Standards Review Council and a consultant to state and federal regulatory agencies on health law issues. She lectures widely on these issues for various organizations including the National Health Lawyers Association, American Medical Association, American Medical Peer Review Association, Blue Cross and Blue Shield Association, and others. A member of the executive committee of the National Health Lawyers Association, she has chaired their programs on utilization management, PROs, and quality assurance and is on the planning committee for their jointly sponsored programs with the American Medical Association on physician legal issues. Ms. Gosfield has published a book on PSROs, numerous articles on utilization management and quality assurance topics, and is a contributing editor of the *1989 Health Law Handbook* and the forthcoming *1990 Health Law Handbook*, published by Clark Boardman Co., Ltd. She is also the consulting editor to Clark Boardman Co., Ltd.'s, health law series. She was a member of the Institute of Medicine Committee on Utilization Management by Third Parties.

MICHAEL A.W. HATTWICK, M.D., is a practicing physician with Woodburn Internal Medicine Associates, Ltd., a five-physician primary care internal medicine practice that he founded in Fairfax County, Virginia, in 1977. He was born in Illinois, raised in Texas, and educated at Harvard, Georgetown, and the University of London. He is board certified in internal medicine and in preventive medicine, with a subspecialty interest in preventive cardiology. He is currently a clinical assistant professor of the Departments of Medicine and Community and Family Medicine of Georgetown University School of Medicine, a member of the governing council of the Virginia chapter of the American College of Physicians, a trustee of the Virginia Society of Internal Medicine, and a member of the American Medical Association. Since 1978, he has been actively using computers to implement preventive medicine guidelines in his clinical practice. Prior to entering full-time medical practice, he served as chief medical advisor and director of the Health Examination Survey of the National Center for Health Statistics, director of the Surveillance and Assessment Center of the National Influenza Immunization Program, director of the Special Pathogens Branch of the Viral Disease Division Epidemiology Program at the Centers for Disease Control, and registrar and visiting lecturer at St. Thomas' Hospital Medical School.

CLARK C. HAVIGHURST, J.D., is William Neal Reynolds Professor of Law at Duke University. He is also professor of community health sciences at the Duke University Medical School. During the 1989-1990 academic year, he was on sabbatical at the firm of Epstein, Becker & Green in Washington, D.C. Mr. Havighurst received his undergraduate degree from Princeton University and his law degree from Northwestern University. He is the author of a leading law school casebook, *Health Care Law and Policy* (Foundation Press, 1988), and *Deregulating the Health Care Industry* (Ballinger, 1982). He will shortly publish a major article on practice guidelines in the *Saint Louis University Law Journal*. His other writings include numerous articles on health insurance, professional liability, and competition and antitrust issues in the health care field. On earlier sabbaticals, he served as consultant to the U.S. Federal Trade Commission (1988-1989) and as a scholar-in-residence at the IOM (1972-1973). He has been an IOM member since 1982.

ADA SUE HINSHAW, Ph.D., R.N., F.A.A.N., has been director of the National Center for Nursing Research at the National Institutes of Health since June 1987. Prior positions included professor and director of research at the University of Arizona College of Nursing while concurrently serving as director of nursing research at University Medical Center. Dr. Hinshaw received her Ph.D. in sociology from the University of Arizona, holds two master's degrees–in sociology, from the University of Arizona, and nursing, from Yale University–and earned her undergraduate degree in nursing from the University of Kansas. Dr. Hinshaw has published widely. Her honorary and professional affiliations include the American Nurses Association, Council of Nurse Researchers, Sigma Xi, American Academy of Nursing, Sigma Theta Tau, Inc., the National Academies of Practice, and the Institute of Medicine. She has conducted numerous extramurally funded studies focused on nursing systems and nursing administration research.

JOHN T. KELLY, M.D., Ph.D., has been director of the American Medical Association's (AMA) Office of Quality Assurance since June 1988. He coordinates the AMA/Specialty Society Practice Parameters Forum and is the editor of the AMA's quality assurance newsletter. Formerly, he was associate medical director of California Medical Review, Inc., the California peer review organization; chairman of the Quality Assurance Committee of the American Medical Peer Review Association; and a practicing emergency physician. He has also served as president of the San Francisco Emergency Physicians Association. He received his undergraduate training from Amherst College, his doctorate in the history of science from Harvard University, and his medical degree from Harvard Medical School. His residency training was in internal medicine and radiology.

DONALD G. LANGSLEY, M.D., is executive vice president of the American Board of Medical Specialties and professor of psychiatry and behavioral sciences at Northwestern University School of Medicine. He was formerly professor and chairman of psychiatry at the University of Cincinnati and, for nine years previously, the first chairman of the Psychiatry Department at the University of California, Davis, School of Medicine. He has also been president of the American Psychiatric Association and of the National Resident Matching Plan. He is a member of the board of trustees of the Educational Commission for Foreign Medical Graduates and a member of the National Board of Medical Examiners. Dr. Langsley was a director of the American Board of Psychiatry and Neurology and a member of the Residency Review Committee in Psychiatry and Neurology.

LAWRENCE C. MORRIS is a consultant in health care finance, based in Wilmette, Illinois. Before becoming a consultant, he spent 23 years with the Blue Cross and Blue Shield Association, the majority of that time as senior vice president for professional affairs and health benefits management. Previously, he was for 10 years executive director of the Medical Society of Delaware. Mr. Morris was an originator of the Blue Cross and Blue Shield Medical Necessity Program, the first collaborative effort among national medical specialty societies and a payment agency to establish guidelines for cost-effective practice. He was a member of the Institute of Medicine's Council on Health Care Technology and chair of its Information Panel.

JOACHIM L. OPITZ, M.D., is professor of physical medicine and rehabilitation, Mayo Medical School, Rochester, Minnesota. His medical degrees are from the University of Goettingen (West Germany) and the University of Minnesota, and he is board certified in physical medicine and rehabilitation. Dr. Opitz has been president of the American Academy of Physical Medicine and Rehabilitation and is its current delegate to the Council of Medical Specialty Societies. Among other professional society activities, he chairs the Task Force on Practice Guidelines and Standards of the American Spinal Injury Association. He is the author of numerous articles in the field of rehabilitation medicine and professional education.

JOHN C. PETERSON III, M.D., is the chairman of the Medical Directors Section of AMPRA, the American Medical Peer Review Association. He is also director of medical affairs for the Professional Review Organization for Washington, Alaska, and Idaho. He has served in that position since 1986. Dr. Peterson has had an active clinical practice in internal medicine and family practice in Seattle, Washington, since 1972 and serves as clinical associate professor of family practice at the University of Washington School of Medicine. Dr. Peterson joined the staff of Northwest Hospital in Seattle, Washington, in 1972, where he has served in various positions, including chairman of the Credentials Committee. He is a fellow of the American Academy of Family Practice and a member of the American College of Physicians.

ELLISON C. PIERCE, JR., M.D., is associate clinical professor of anaesthesia at Harvard Medical School and chairman of the Department of Anaesthesia at the New England Deaconess Hospital. He was the 1984 president of the American Society of Anesthesiologists and is a current chairman of its Committee on Patient Safety and Risk Management. In 1985 he founded and became president of the Anesthesia Patient Safety Foundation, a multidisciplinary organization dedicated to all facets of patient safety in anesthesia. Dr. Pierce is chairman of the Task Force on Practice Policies of the Council of Medical Specialty Societies, a member of the American Medical Association Practice Parameters Forum, a member of the Joint Commission of Anesthesia Care's Clinical Indicator Task Force, and a member of the World Federation of Societies of Anesthesiologists' Committee on Safety in Anaesthesia. He is an authority on anesthesia patient safety and risk management and has lectured and written on anesthesia in the diabetic patient, the medical liability crisis, and patient safety and risk management. Dr. Pierce is president and chief executive officer of Anaesthesia Associates of Boston, P.C., a group practice providing services to two major Boston teaching hospitals and several other Massachusetts hospitals and surgicenters.

BRENDA RICHARDSON, M.D., is a practicing physician in Massachusetts. She is the president of the Massachusetts Peer Review Organization, a wholly owned subsidiary of the Massachusetts Medical Society. Dr. Richardson graduated from McMaster Medical School and the Harvard School of Public Health. In addition to her PRO activities, she maintains a consulting practice in nutrition, is the school physician for the city of Gloucester, and is the medical director of quality assurance and utilization review at the Addison-Gilbert Hospital in Gloucester, Massachusetts. Dr. Richardson is board certified by the American Board of Quality Assurance and Utilization Review Physicians. She is a past president of the local chapter of the American Cancer Society and a current member of the Professional Advisory Board of the Visiting Nurses Association of the North Shore.

LOUISE RUSSELL, Ph.D., is research professor of economics at the Institute for Health, Health Care Policy, and Aging Research, Rutgers University, and a professor in the Department of Economics. Before joining Rutgers in 1987, Dr. Russell was a senior fellow at the Brookings Institution for 12 years. Her most recent Brookings book is *Medicare's New Hospital Payment System: Is It Working?* (1989), an evaluation of the success of Medicare's DRG-based payment rates for hospitals. Her Brookings publications also include *Evaluating Preventive Care: Report on a Workshop* (1987), *Is Prevention Better Than Cure?* (1986), *The Baby Boom Generation and the Economy* (1982), and *Technology in Hospitals: Medical Advances and Their Diffusion* (1979). She has written numerous journal articles as well as chapters in several editions of Brookings' regular volumes on the federal budget. Dr. Russell is a member of the Institute of Medicine. She served on the Institute's Committee for the Study of the Future of Public Health (1986-1987) and currently serves on its Board on Health Sciences Policy. She was also a member of the U.S. Preventive Services Task Force of the Department of Health and Human Services (1984-1988).

WILLIAM STASON, M.D., M.S., received his M.D. degree, cum laude, from the Harvard Medical School in 1960 and his master of science degree in epidemiology from the Harvard School of Public Health in 1975. He trained in internal medicine and cardiology at the Massachusetts General Hospital, Boston, Massachusetts, and Columbia Presbyterian Hospital, New York, New York. He has been a member of the Harvard faculty since 1970 and is currently lecturer in health policy and management at the Harvard School of Public Health and lecturer in medicine at the Harvard Medical School. For the past 20 years, Dr. Stason has been involved in planning, managing, and evaluating health care services. He is currently director of the Department of Veterans Affairs Northeast Health Services Research and Development Field Program located at the West Roxbury, Massachusetts, Medical Center and vice president of Health Economics Research, Inc., of Needham, Massachusetts.

MICHAEL A. STOCKER, M.D., M.P.H., has been executive vice president and general manager of the Greater New York Marketplace since May 1989 and senior vice president and general manager of the Greater New York Marketplace since July 1987. Since November 1986 he has been president of U.S. Healthcare, Inc. (New York), and from October 1985 to October 1986 he was vice president and medical director of the same subsidiary. From 1980 to 1985 he was medical director of the Anchor Organization for Health Maintenance of the Rush Presbyterian St. Luke's Medical Center in Chicago. Prior to that he was associate chairman of the Department of Family Practice at Cook County Hospital in Chicago from 1975 to 1980. Dr. Stocker was educated at the University of Notre Dame and received his M.D. degree from the Medical College of Wisconsin in 1968. He received his postgraduate training at the Mayo Clinic and the University of California, Davis, and is board certified in internal medicine and family practice. Dr. Stocker also received a master's degree in public health from the University of Michigan in 1978.

JAMES J. STRAIN, M.D., is professor and director of the Division of Behavioral Medicine and Consultation Psychiatry at the Mount Sinai School of Medicine. He is president of the Society of Liaison Psychiatry, co-chairman of the MICRO-CARES Consultation/Liaison Consortium for computerized data management systems and collaborative studies, and scientific advisor to the European Consultation/Liaison Work Group. He is a former chairperson of ethics at the Mount Sinai School of Medicine. Under National Institute of Mental Health contracts and grants, he has pioneered models of mental health training for primary care physicians and cost-offset evaluation for psychiatric interventions in the medical setting. Funded by the National Cancer Institute, he has developed models to examine physician adherence to protocols and thereby provided schema